S0-BXG-749

FROM A GYNECOLOGIST'S NOTEBOOK

By Sherwin A. Kaufman, M.D.

THE AGELESS WOMAN

NEW HOPE FOR THE CHILDLESS COUPLE

FROM A GYNECOLOGIST'S NOTEBOOK

QUESTIONS WOMEN ASK

SHERWIN A. KAUFMAN, M.D.

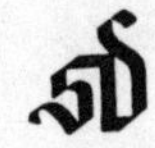

STEIN AND DAY/*Publishers*/New York

First published in 1974

Library of Congress Catalog Card No. 74-79423

Designed by David Miller
Printed in the United States of America
Stein and Day/*Publishers*/Scarborough House, Briarcliff Manor, N.Y. 10510
ISBN 08128-1706-0

To those I love—
my wife, Claire,
and my sons,
Kenneth, Keith, and Michael

Contents

Introduction

When I was a youngster, all medical questions were referred to "the doctor in the house," my father, who seemed to have a limitless reservoir of knowledge on any topic, based on his many years as a general practitioner. I can remember the comfortable feeling of knowing that whatever the problem, there was always an answer.

But that was many years ago, in a very personal setting. It was also before the days of "superspecialization," resulting from the steady advances in medical science.

Actually, no speciality stands alone. The obstetrician-gynecologist must frequently draw upon his knowledge of other fields to arrive at a proper diagnosis. By the same token, often it is the family physician, the internist, or the surgeon who is suddenly called upon to answer such questions as are found in this book. Frequently, consultation is required, so that the closest cooperation between the various specialties is essential. Of course, the answers I propose are not meant to replace your doctor's advice.

This book evolved from three different sources.

First, it is a natural outgrowth of my question-and-answer column which has appeared in various editions of *Family Circle* Magazine over the past five years. The column, called "What Does the Doctor Say?" responds to letters from women throughout the country, about various gynecological and obstetrical subjects. In fact, many questions in this book have appeared in *Family Circle.* Many more have remained unanswered until now, due to limitations in magazine space.

It is evident from these letters that many women are reluctant to consult a gynecologist even when they have specific complaints. Many are obviously too embarrassed to inquire about their problem in their own community, preferring the anonymity of a letter. The accumulated mound of correspondence indicates a hunger for straightforward information apparently not easily (or comfortably) available nearer home. Every age group is represented—the adolescent, the young single, the young married, the maturing woman, the woman in menopause, and the elderly.

A second source of material for this book comes from my experience as Medical Director of Planned Parenthood in the New York area for over twenty years. This includes seven years with Planned Parenthood of New York City, which treats almost 50,000 patients a year. This agency provides a wide range of family planning services and conducts major training and educational programs.

The third source for this book comes from my more than twenty-five years in the private practice of gynecology and obstetrics. In contrast to years ago, when "personal" matters had to be carefully drawn out, I find that nowadays women are likely to volunteer such information without hesitation, in line with the more relaxed, almost casual air of frankness about gynecological, marital, and sexual problems.

In the privacy of the consultation room over the past twenty-five years, the many queries from countless women have encompassed every aspect of QUESTIONS WOMEN ASK.

Sherwin A. Kaufman, M.D.

ONE

Reproductive Riddles

Dear Dr. Kaufman:

Of the total number of sperm in an ejaculation, about how many reach the area of the tube that contains the egg?

Answer:

It is estimated that only several thousand of the 400 to 500 million produced reach the tube.

Dear Dr. Kaufman:

How rapidly can a sperm travel?

Answer:

Under ideal conditions, a sperm can swim about one inch in 6-8 minutes. However, since it does not always swim in a straight line, it often takes much longer to go an inch. Incidentally, the length of the cervical canal is just about one inch.

Dear Dr. Kaufman:

How large is a human sperm?

Answer:

The total length of a sperm, from the top of its "head" to the tip of its "tail" is about 1/600 inch. The oval head itself is 1/6,000 inch in diameter. Thus the tail is ten times as long as the head.

Dear Dr. Kaufman:

Does each ovary produce an egg each month, on an alternate basis?

Answer:

No. Apparently the ovaries accomplish this without a definite plan. Sometimes they do alternate, but at other times the same ovary might release an egg a few months in a row.

Dear Dr. Kaufman:

What is double ovulation?

Answer:

It is the release of more than one egg at a time, and this is the way non-identical twins are conceived.

Dear Dr. Kaufman:

I have heard an expression that birth is an accident of fate. Could you explain the meaning?

Answer:

It probably refers to the fact that at the moment of conception, only one of perhaps a half billion sperm has a chance of becoming your biological father. No two of these half billion sperm are exactly alike, each having a slightly different chromosomal (blueprint) makeup. In your case, if any other one of those half billion sperm had fertilized the ovum from which you were born, you would have been an entirely different person!

Dear Dr. Kaufman:

When does an embryo become a fetus?

Answer:

By definition the embryo has grown to a fetus by the end of the second month. It then measures about one inch and weighs 1/30th of an ounce.

Dear Dr. Kaufman:

I understand that after ejaculation, the sperm swim up and some reach the tube. What if there is no egg released yet?

Answer:

The more patient sperm will just cruise in the tube, waiting for the release of the egg. If it is released within three days or so, it is still possible for fertilization to take place.

Dear Dr. Kaufman:

How large is the human egg?

Answer:

The ovum is about 1/200 inch in diameter—approximately ¼ the size of a punctuation dot.

Dear Dr. Kaufman:

How deep is the vagina? I am 24, built quite normally, but have difficulty with intercourse.

Answer:

Once the hymen is passed, difficulty with intercourse is not due to being "small" but rather to tension or fear causing tightening of the muscles around the vagina. The vagina itself measures about 3¾ inches and is readily stretchable.

Dear Dr. Kaufman:

Is the egg of a whale much larger than that of a human?

Answer:

No. The egg of a whale is not a whale of an egg. It is not much larger than a human egg.

Dear Dr. Kaufman:

If it takes only one sperm to fertilize an egg, why are so many millions needed to begin with? I also understand that hundreds are needed just to have one penetrate.

Answer:

The process of "sperm meets egg" is not as simple as it sounds. In order to complete the genetic union, it is necessary for the sperm to first penetrate the egg's outer coating. To do this, the sperm is equipped with a special chemical. The necessity of softening the egg's covering may be one reason why so many hundreds of sperm are in the neighborhood. Even so, it is not known how only one sperm manages to gain complete entry, but it is believed that it takes advantage of the softening action of the other sperm around it.

Dear Dr. Kaufman:

How long do sperm survive in the body after intercourse? For how long is an ovum capable of being fertilized?

Answer:

In the *vagina* sperm survive for only a short time—a very few hours at the most. Many sperm are killed almost immediately by the normally hostile vaginal secretions. However, once sperm gain entrance into the cervix, where the secretion is more favorable, they can continue their ascent and are capable of fertilizing an egg for about two or three days. Some sperm may survive in the female reproductive tract for a week or more, but their ability to fertilize an egg diminishes with time.

The ovum is capable of being fertilized for about one or two days after being extruded.

Thus, the total fertile period, taking into account the number of days during which sperm can retain their ability to fertilize and the ovum retains the capacity to be fertilized, probably does not exceed three or four days. The real difficulty is in pinpointing which days they will be.

Dear Dr. Kaufman:

After intercourse, how long does it take the sperm to reach the Fallopian tube where fertilization takes place?

Answer:

Estimates vary from thirty minutes to three hours.

Dear Dr. Kaufman:

I would be interested in knowing the derivation of common words dealing with the sexual and reproductive organs of women.

Answer:

Vulva means "covering" in Latin; it is the collective name for the entire group of female external genital organs.

Hymen is the name of the mythical God of Marriage.

Mons Veneris means the "Mount of Venus" and is the cushion of fat over the pubis, covered with hair and protecting the inner organs of reproduction.

Clitoris means "that which is closed in" in Latin. This erotic organ is literally closed in by a fold of tissue.

Vagina means "sheath" in Latin.

Cervix means "neck" in Latin, referring to the neck of the uterus.

Uterus means "belly" or "womb" in Latin.

Ovaries means "egg-aries," from the Latin word ova, which means egg.

Oviducts means "egg ducts." They are also known as Fallopian tubes after the 16th-century physician Gregario Fallopio, who erroneously thought they were "ventilators" for the uterus.

Dear Dr. Kaufman:

Although it may sound like a silly question, I would like to know if it is possible for me to get pregnant if I have my underclothes on. I am really worried about it.

Answer:

It would require considerable seepage of semen through the garment at the vaginal entrance. While not very likely that this would result in pregnancy, it is a possibility and has actually happened.

Dear Dr. Kaufman:

How is it possible for a woman to become pregnant if she has sex relations during her menstrual period only? This has happened to a friend of mine, and I know she is telling me the truth.

Answer:

There are several ways. The most likely possibility is that an egg was released unusually early that particular cycle—say on the seventh day. The woman could then conceive by having intercourse on the 4th, 5th, or 6th day of her cycle–that is, during her menstrual period. Had she *not* conceived that cycle, her next period would have come unusually early (about 21 days rather than 28), due to the unusually early ovulation.

Another possibility, which is more likely in women who are irregular and whose menstrual periods are relatively light, is that she mistook ovulation staining for a period. In that event, she would be having intercourse at the most fertile, rather than the least fertile time of the month.

Another possibility, though less likely, is that ovulation was induced by the very act of intercourse.

Dear Dr. Kaufman:

I have had five boys, and very much want a girl. Is it true that there is a tendency to produce a preponderance of males in some families (or vice versa)? If so, should I just give up trying?

Answer:

Investigations by geneticists and statisticians indicate that the production of a child of one sex or the other is not affected by heredity. The sex of an infant appears to be purely a matter of chance.

You may recall the old coin-tossing experiments. You will get 7 heads or 7 tails in a row once in 128 tosses. What this means is that your chances of having a boy in your next pregnancy are the same whether you have already had five sons or five daughters.

Actually, many more boys are *conceived* than girls, but the much higher male intrauterine death rate results in a final birth ratio which is almost equal—106 boys to 100 girls.

Dear Dr. Kaufman:

Who determines the sex of the baby? Is it the mother or the father?

Answer:

It is the father who determines the baby's sex. The female egg is neutral. The male sperm carries either an X or a Y chromosome. If an X-chromosome-carrying sperm fertilizes the egg, it will be a girl, but if a Y-sperm meets the egg first, a boy will be the result.

Dear Dr. Kaufman:

I understand that the sex of a child can be determined, after pregnancy has been initiated, by studying the fluid surrounding the baby. How is this done?

Answer:

The sex of the fetus can be predicted before birth in the following manner: About 10 cc of fluid surrounding the fetus are drawn and after special processing, fetal cells are stained and studied. A boy is predicted if the sex chromatin count is less than three per cent, a girl if it is twelve per cent or more.

Dear Dr. Kaufman:

Can knowing the sex of a baby before it is born be of value for medical purposes?

Answer:

Yes, knowing the sex of the baby prenatally can help diagnose such sex-linked hereditary diseases as hemophilia, childhood muscular dystrophy, congenital adrenal hyperplasia, and mongolism. On the other hand, the method of withdrawing amniotic fluid for such studies is not meant to simply satisfy the curiosity of parents concerning the sex of the unborn baby, since the procedure is not without danger to the mother and fetus.

Dear Dr. Kaufman:

Can the odds be changed as to whether you might have a boy or a girl?

Answer:

From time to time, some investigators have thought—and some still do—that the odds can be significantly changed. One theory, based on clinical impressions and insemination cases holds that the sex of the baby is determined by the time of conception in relation to ovulation; that there are more female births when conception takes place either more than 48 hours before ovulation or 10 hours after ovulation; and that male births are favored by conception very close to ovulation.

However, other research specifically designed to test this hypothesis did not come up with the same findings and failed to substantiate the theory—that is, no predictable relationship was found between the time of conception and the sex of the baby. In still another study, donor insemination close to ovulation resulted in a preponderance of male offspring, whereas husband insemination close to ovulation resulted paradoxically in a preponderance of female offspring.

One researcher has advanced the theory that male-producing sperm (bearing the Y chromosome) are smaller and faster moving than female-bearing sperm, which supposedly are larger and sturdier, better able to fertilize an egg that does not arrive for two or three days. This observer claims to be able to distinguish male-bearing from female-bearing sperm microscopically. For those desiring a boy, he advises a bicarbonate (alkaline) douche before intercourse, to coincide with ovulation, with prior abstention. For a girl, he favors a vinegar (acid) douche before intercourse, timed about two days before expected ovulation. It should be added that the same conclusions have not been reached by several other researchers, who have found no decisive evidence that male-bearing and female-bearing sperm are different in size and shape, or that they can be distinguished microscopically or separated from each other. Also, it should be mentioned that timing of ovulation is very difficult and imprecise.

Dear Dr. Kaufman:

Unfortunately, the only child I have had was a mongoloid. I wondered what advances have been made in genetics that might prevent this kind of "accident" from occurring.

Answer:

The English scientist, Lord C.P. Snow, quotes his friend Charles Scribner, Jr., as observing: "God deals one a hand of cards, and all education can do is to teach one how best to play it." At the same time, Lord Snow observes that although humans are not born equal (that is, not born with equal genetic endowment, either physical, intellectual, or temperamental), yet in a deeper sense human beings are born equal in that they are born to live, endure, and die. It may well be that *genetic engineering* may some day be able to completely eradicate such gross genetic "misinstruction" as the one that produced a mongoloid in your case and doubtless has caused you much suffering.

Genetics is a relatively new and fascinating field. Normally, every body cell has 46 chromosomes, containing hundreds of pairs of genes arranged in twisting strands of tiny programmed computers containing all the instructions for dictating the size and shape of every organ. One gene in each pair is inherited from the father and is matched with a gene having the same function, inherited from the mother. Such matching must be superb, considering the relative paucity of defects.

When genetic defects do occur, it might be because an abnormal recessive gene happened to be matched with another abnormal recessive gene just like it; if a dominant gene is abnormal, the defect will develop regardless of the matching gene. Other causes of genetic defects are various virus infections or the use of certain drugs during early pregnancy. Mutations may also follow irradiation, or have completely obscure causes.

Dear Dr. Kaufman:

I have always had a morbid fear of having an abnormal child. What are the odds?

Answer:

In humans, the incidence of fetal anomalies is greatest when reproductive life is just beginning (in the teen-ager), and again when it is almost over (women in their forties). The incidence of such anomalies is about 2 per cent at age 15; it falls to less than 1 per cent during reproductive life; after age 35 it again slowly increases, to above 2 per cent in the forties.

Dear Dr. Kaufman:

Since a true hermaphrodite possesses both male and female sex organs, is it possible for self-impregnation to occur?

Answer:

In most cases, the external genitals of a true hermaphrodite most nearly resemble the male, and indeed most are reared as males. However, the structure of the internal genitals varies greatly, and it is unusual for totally male and female ducts to be simultaneously present.

It is possible for both the male and female sex gland tissue to be hormonally active at different times, as is evidenced by the development of male external genitals at birth, followed by breast development and menstruation after the onset of puberty. Although testicular tissue after puberty is usually nonfunctioning, occasional cases of sperm production concurrent with menstruation have been observed. However, no true hermaphrodites have ever been known to "reproduce" and they are considered to be clinically infertile.

TWO

Pregnancy and Childbirth

Dear Dr. Kaufman:

What is the earliest possible diagnostic test for pregnancy?

Answer:

If a woman has been keeping her basal temperature record, this will give an early clue. A 20-day sustained elevation after ovulation, in the absence of illness, is considered a positive sign of pregnancy with a very high degree of accuracy.

Earlier still are some new, complex blood tests which make it possible to diagnose pregnancy even before a menstrual period is missed. Such tests utilize laboratory techniques known as "radio-immune," or "radio-receptor assays."

Dear Dr. Kaufman:

I am intrigued by the rapidity with which modern tests can detect the presence or absence of pregnancy in a few minutes. How do these tests work?

Answer:

Such pregnancy tests rely on the presence of a certain hormone in the urine called chorionic gonadotropin, manufactured by the placenta. Enough of it appears within 10-14 days after a missed period to give a positive pregnancy test in most instances.

The "original" pregnancy test was described by Drs. Selmar Ascheim and Bernhardt Zondek in 1928 (the AZ test). Urine was injected into a young female mouse, and the ovaries were examined about 100 hours later. In 1931 a modification of the AZ test was introduced by Dr. Maurice H. Friedman and Dr. Maxwell E. Lapham (the Friedman test), reducing the time from five days to two days, and using rabbits instead of mice (the "rabbit test").

More recently, immunological procedures have been used, and these are the quick slide tests you have referred to. A drop of the woman's urine is mixed with a drop of antiserum, then the combination is mixed with two drops of hormone-coated latex particles. Within 2-3 minutes, the verdict is known. Besides being quick, this test has the advantage of not requiring animals or incubators, and can be done in the doctor's office with a minimum of equipment.

Dear Dr. Kaufman:

What produces so-called false positive pregnancy tests in the absence of pregnancy?

Answer:

False positive pregnancy tests may occur if there is an extended time interval between collecting the urine and doing the test; when there is a large protein excretion in the urine; when certain tranquilizers are ingested; and during menopause. But the most frequent cause may be a simple laboratory error.

Dear Dr. Kaufman:

How can a woman tell for sure if she's pregnant? I have heard that pregnancy tests are not infallible and that often a doctor can't be sure either. Are there any absolute tests?

Answer:

The only 100% absolute tests are: hearing the fetal heart, feeling fetal movements, and x-ray (or ultrasound). Unfortunately, except for ultrasound, these indicators don't appear till the woman is several months along. However, there are some very good presumptive signs of pregnancy that show up very early. The missing of a period is, of course, important. A positive pregnancy test is about 95 per cent accurate, provided the woman is at least 10-12 days late due to pregnancy. And, of course, there are many clues on examination—a softened, enlarged uterus, bluish discoloration of the cervix, congested breasts, frequent urination, fatigue, and nausea.

Dear Dr. Kaufman:

When I had my baby ten years ago, my husband almost went to pieces in the "father's room," pacing the floor for hours. I understand there has been a trend to involve the husband more actively. Is this only in the larger hospital centers or throughout the country?

Answer:

Pretty much throughout the country. Husbands are indeed encouraged to participate during their wife's labor and even delivery, and special classes are given widely to prepare the expectant parents for what is to come.

Dear Dr. Kaufman:

I am curious to know: statistically, how much does a Caesarean section increase the risk of maternal death?

Answer:

The over-all maternal mortality rate in the United States is about 24 per 100,000 live births, or 2.4 per 10,000 live births. Caesarean section today, even in the best of hands, carries a mortality rate of 2 per 1,000 or 20 per 10,000. Stating it another way, the maternal death risk of Caesarean section is about eight times higher than the over-all maternal mortality. Of course, it should be kept in mind that Caesarean section is often done in inherently difficult situations of an emergency nature.

Dear Dr. Kaufman:

Is the term "Caesarean section" named after Julius Caesar?

Answer:

No, Caesar had a normal birth; but an early ancestor, Scipio Africanus, was born by Caesarean. He was thence dubbed the "cut out one" (in Latin, "Caesar"). Incidentally, the word can be spelled either Caesarean or cesarean.

Dear Dr. Kaufman:

I was wondering how it is that women of small build and stature manage to give birth normally. I would think that most would need to have Caesareans. Can you explain?

Answer:

A "small" woman does not necessarily have a small pelvis. It is the configuration of the pelvic bones that determines the amount of room. Much also depends upon the size of the baby and the force of uterine contractions.

Years ago, I became particularly interested in the very question you pose, and made a study of the narrowest portion of the bony pelvis (called the midpelvis) in "small" women, in relation to the kind of labor and delivery they had. The study was published in a medical journal, under what had to be one of the longest titles in medical annals: "A Consideration of the Midpelvis Among the Factors which may Influence the Course and Outcome of Labor." In any event, I found surprisingly few problem cases. Most of the women with small pelves overcame this handicap by superior force of contractions, and the "anticipated" high Caesarean rate did not materialize.

Dear Dr. Kaufman:

I am three months' pregnant and this is my first baby. Although there is a hospital near my home, the obstetrician and hospital I would prefer to go to for my delivery are over an hour away. Should I be concerned?

Answer:

No. While getting to the hospital on time is a common worry (husbands worry even more), there is plenty of time for the first baby. In fact, you can anticipate many hours of labor with more than enough time to get to the hospital in leisure. The rather dramatic mad dashes, or deliveries by taxi drivers that you hear or read about in the newspapers almost always involve women who have had several babies, with a history of progressively shorter labors with each.

Dear Dr. Kaufman:

I am in my second month of pregnancy, and am confused by advice from several different sources as to the safety of taking any common drugs such as aspirin, tranquilizers, sleeping pills, etc. Can you clarify this for me?

Answer:

You do not state your "sources"—whether articles in popular journals, friends, relatives, or (presumably) your doctor. In any event, to answer your question, there seems to be a consensus of medical opinion that the fewer drugs taken during early pregnancy, the better. This is not to say that taking any of the items you mention is necessarily "dangerous" but simply that early embryonic and fetal physiology is so complex that it is far simpler to avoid any unnecessary drugs than to interpolate animal studies regarding possible harmful effects. The key word here is "unnecessary." There are special situations where certain drugs are quite essential for some particular condition. If that's the case, your doctor will undoubtedly advise you accordingly. One must always weigh the benefits against the potential risks.

Dear Dr. Kaufman:

During the early weeks of my first pregnancy I had much pelvic discomfort, but my obstetrician assured me that the baby was growing quite normally. He was apparently right, since I recently was delivered of a healthy little girl. Looking back, could you explain why there should have been so much discomfort during those first few weeks?

Answer:

It is common, especially during the early part of the first pregnancy, to feel pelvic discomfort; this has been ascribed usually to the stretching of the uterus and surrounding tissues. There is generally also some apprehension connected with the first pregnancy that may contribute to, or accentuate such discomfort. Reassurance was the proper treatment.

Dear Dr. Kaufman:

Is there any objection to a long car ride during early pregnancy? Plane travel?

Answer:

Not if the pregnancy is a normal one, as far as can be determined by the history and the physical examination.

Dear Dr. Kaufman:

In the United States, what is the actual risk of death from pregnancy and childbirth?

Answer:

The risk of death from pregnancy and delivery (exclusive of death from illegal abortion) in the 20 to 34 age group is 23 per 100,000. In the age group 35 to 44, the risk rises to three times that rate.

Dear Dr. Kaufman:

Can a woman conceive after she has already become pregnant? Would this cause twins?

Answer:

Conceiving again after pregnancy (so-called superfetation) does not take place in humans. Fraternal twins are caused by the almost simultaneous fertilization of two eggs by two different sperm, but I don't think your question referred to that. Identical twins are produced when a single fertilized egg splits into two, and each develops into a separate embryo.

Dear Dr. Kaufman:

What determines whether a woman will have twins? My doctor suspects that I will have two babies, but there are no twins on my side of the family or my husband's.

Answer:

Twins occur in one out of 90 pregnancies. Whether or not a woman is likely to bear twins depends on certain predisposing factors: her age, race, the number of children she has already had, and her hereditary background. Statistically speaking, a woman has a greater chance of having twins if she is older (but not past 40), black, has had several children, or if there are twins in her family or in her husband's. However, such predisposing factors apply only to fraternal (two egg) twins. Identical twins, which occur much less commonly, are not dependent on such factors, and seem to be a matter of pure chance. (Of course, these statistical predispositons do not include women taking fertility drugs.)

Dear Dr. Kaufman:

A lot of my friends had trouble with breast engorgement after delivery. What can be done to prevent this kind of discomfort?

Answer:

Breast engorgement after delivery, for the mother who chooses not to nurse, is best treated by prevention. For this purpose, estrogen, progesterone, testosterone, or a combination of these may be used. Some doctors use no medication at all except mild analgesics if needed.

Prevention of milk engorgement is optimal when medication is given well before lactation begins. The suppressive drugs should be continued long enough for a smooth transition, and also to minimize chances of delayed engorgement after the medication is discontinued.

Relatively small doses of estrogen, given for seven to ten days, starting the day of delivery, usually prevents this problem satisfactorily. Some doctors prefer testosterone, the male sex hormone, either orally or as an injectable, combined with a long-acting estrogen.

Dear Dr. Kaufman:

I have decided after a great deal of thought to try to breast-feed my baby, but I am very worried I may not be able to. I have heard that a mother's emotional state may affect her capacity to produce milk. How can I be sure I will be able to breast-feed my baby, which is what I want so much to do?

Answer:

You should make it clearly known to your doctor and to just about everyone you come into contact with at the hospital that you intend to breast-feed, so that there is no misunderstanding. The cooperation of the hospital staff is most important, and the key to the whole procedure is to make sure the baby is brought to the breast at regular intervals (this will stimulate the onset of milk production). It must be equally clear that the nursery is not to do you the "favor" of giving the baby any formulas in order to let you "rest," since this can torpedo your success rate for breast-feeding.

Ideally, the baby should receive its milk exclusively from the breast, and it would be most helpful if your doctor leaves explicit orders with the nursery to this effect so that no well-meaning personnel can undermine your wishes. Most hospitals will gladly cooperate if you make known your desires in this matter.

Dear Dr. Kaufman:

All my friends, even those who haven't had children, insist that breast-feeding is much better for the child than bottle-feeding. I have a job which interests me very much, and I would like to be able to get back to at least part-time work after my baby is born. I want to do the best for my baby, but are my friends right when they say that if I feed the baby by the bottle I will be hurting him in some way?

Answer:

Your so-called "friends" are doing you no favor in making you feel guilty about your intent to bottle-feed your baby. While there is no denying the value of breast milk, which is the ideal nutrient, keep in mind that countless millions of infants have been bottle-fed and have thrived beautifully! I have found that a reluctant breast-feeder is rarely a successful breast-feeder anyway, so gain comfort in the knowledge that you will not be "harming" your baby by bottle-feeding.

Dear Dr. Kaufman:

Can I become pregnant while nursing? I have heard conflicting reports about this.

Answer:

You have very little chance of becoming pregnant while nursing until the baby is 10 weeks old—unless you have a menstrual period before that time, which is unlikely. After the baby is 10 weeks old, the chance of conception gradually increases.

Dear Dr. Kaufman:

Does the size of the breasts have a relationship to the ability to nurse? Mine are rather small, and I am expecting my baby in about five months.

Answer:

No, the size of a mother's breasts has nothing to do with her ability to nurse her baby. The glandular mechanism responsible for nursing is independent of breast size. The vast majority of women are able to nurse if they so desire, regardless of breast size.

Dear Dr. Kaufman:

If drugs are taken by a nursing mother, are they transmitted to the baby?

Answer:

A great many drugs are capable of being transmitted to an infant via breast milk, but they are usually present in such small amounts that they produce no symptoms in the baby. Aspirin is occasionally responsible for a mild rash in a breast-fed baby and, indeed, many other drugs may be responsible for rashes. Even some unfavorable elements of coffee and tea may be excreted in the mother's milk.

Dear Dr. Kaufman:

I am expecting my first baby and am very much interested in breast-feeding. However, many of my friends are discouraging me, saying that I will develop sore nipples, abscesses, and will be generally tied down. Can you give me good reasons for breast-feeding?

Answer:

A mother who breast-feeds should want to do it. As far as "reasons" are concerned, mother's milk is obviously convenient (no messy or intricate formulas to prepare), and is always readily available at just the right temperature when the baby gets hungry. Breast-fed babies receive special protection against infections because of natural antibodies found in mother's milk. They suffer far less from allergies and serious digestive upsets. Constipation is not a problem as it sometimes is with formula-fed babies.

Dear Dr. Kaufman:

How would you compare human milk with feeding formulas?

Answer:

In contrast to formulas, human milk is always germ free, easier to digest, causes fewer gastro-intestinal upsets, and contains more iron, vitamins, and milk fat. Cow's milk protein may occasionally cause allergies.

Breast milk contains less casein than cow's milk and therefore curdles better. The curd does not remain as long in the stomach, allowing faster digestion.

Dear Dr. Kaufman:

Is it necessary to "prepare" the breasts before delivery if the mother plans to nurse her baby?

Answer:

Although many doctors advise massaging the nipples during the last few weeks of pregnancy to "toughen them up," in my experience the nursing mother does as well without special massage.

Dear Dr. Kaufman:

What is done if a nursing mother's nipples become cracked or sore?

Answer:

Frequently the application of a soothing ointment helps to overcome sore nipples. In more severe cases a special plastic nipple "shield" may be used. If these measures don't help, it may be necessary to stop nursing.

Dear Dr. Kaufman:

I have noticed fairly strong uterine contractions every time I breast-fed my baby. Has this principle ever been used to stimulate the onset of labor?

Answer:

Yes, it has been known and used for a great many years. Stimulation of the nipple by methods such as a suction cup or breast pump can sometimes trigger the release of a special hormone from the pituitary gland and result in uterine contractions. It is especially useful when other methods of stimulation, such as direct hormonal injection or letting out the bag of waters, are considered medically unsuitable. However, breast stimulation is effective only when the uterus is "ready" for labor.

Dear Dr. Kaufman:

Is it safe for a woman in early pregnancy to have dental x-rays? The opinions I get are conflicting.

Answer:

Generally speaking, routine dental x-rays do not directly reach a fetus; any exposure is almost always due to so-called scattered radiation. Although such exposure is extremely small, its further reduction is possible and advisable by the use of a leaded apron shield.

Dear Dr. Kaufman:

What are "afterpains"? Why do some women have them and others do not?

Answer:

So-called afterpains are contractions of the womb during the few days following childbirth. Most first-time mothers are not bothered by afterpains. However, after a second or third baby, the mother is more likely to feel them because there is more loss of muscle tone. Nursing mothers are particularly aware of afterpains, as the infant's sucking stimulates the uterus to contract.

Dear Dr. Kaufman:

I am pregnant and troubled by morning nausea. My doctor is reluctant to prescribe a drug. Is there anything else I can do? I'd like to keep my job till the sixth month.

Answer:

"Morning sickness" (which is not always confined to the morning hours) seldom lasts longer than three months. Try eating some dry crackers before getting out of bed, and wait about 20 minutes after eating the crackers before actually arising. Don't drink fluids right away—liquids often make matters worse. For the rest of the day, try not to let your stomach get empty; have small quantities of food and liquids (together) every hour on the hour.

Dear Dr. Kaufman:

Why aren't all women urged to get the new German measles vaccine, rather than just children? From what I understand, the danger of German measles is to the fetus in a pregnant woman who has contracted the disease.

Answer:

It is important to protect girls against the disease prior to reaching childbearing age. The only hesitancy about giving the vaccine to women of childbearing age is that they might be in an early stage of pregnancy at the time of the vaccination or shortly afterward. Scientists are not sure if the weakened virus in the vaccine will produce the same defects in the embryo as the disease itself. Therefore, the vaccine should be given to adult women only if they are known to be using a reliable contraceptive method and agree to avoid conception for at least 2-3 months following the vaccination.

Dear Dr. Kaufman:

I've heard about ultrasound or sonography and its application in obstetrics and gynecology, and wondered exactly how it works.

Answer:

Ultrasound is a form of mechanical vibrational energy whose frequency is above the normally audible limit of 20,000 cycles per second, ranging instead from 1 million to

10 million cycles per second. At those levels, sound waves can be focused into nearly parallel beams capable of penetrating body tissues. Such sonographic information is reproduced as "blips," which are then converted into a row of luminous dots that form a two-dimensional picture.

Its use in obstetrics, for example, allows positive identification of an early intrauterine pregnancy from the fifth week on, with results immediately available. It can help to clarify the cause of bleeding in early pregnancy and thus facilitate the clinical management of threatened abortion. It can clarify why there might be a discrepancy between the actual uterine size and the size as expected from the last menstrual period. It can corroborate the presence of ovarian cysts, determine the amount of amniotic fluid, and plot the position of the placenta. It can also indicate malposition of the fetus and detect certain anomalies.

In gynecology, sonography can differentiate cystic from solid masses, and establish the presence or absence of an intrauterine device.

Dear Dr. Kaufman:

What advances have been made in monitoring the fetal heart during labor?

Answer:

There are electronic devices which "bug" the fetus by simultaneously monitoring the fetal heart rate and uterine contractions. Although such intensive surveillance has been confined mostly to high risk pregnancies, it is hoped that it may in time be extended to all women in labor in simplified form.

Dear Dr. Kaufman:

I was overweight before conceiving. How much can I expect to lose after the birth of my baby?

Answer:

No matter how much you have gained before childbirth, you can expect to lose about 15 pounds after your baby is born. This represents the combined weight of the baby, the afterbirth, and the amniotic fluid.

Dear Dr. Kaufman:

Is it true that a fast fetal heart rate means a girl baby and a slow one favors a boy?

Answer:

It is true 50 per cent of the time.

Dear Dr. Kaufman:

Must the pregnant woman "eat for two" as the saying goes?

Answer:

No, not for two, but an increase in caloric intake of about 10 per cent over non-pregnant requirements is needed in normal pregnancy to permit the necessary adjustments in maternal physiology and to provide for fetal development. An average total weight gain of about 25 pounds appears to be optimal, according to recent investigation. In evaluating excessive weight gain during pregnancy, it is important to differentiate between fluid retention and actual tissue weight.

Dear Dr. Kaufman:

We have substituted oral-genital contact for sexual intercourse because I am in my last few weeks of pregnancy and I have read that intercourse can sometimes bring on an early birth. I have already had one premature birth. I would appreciate your comments.

Answer:

It is not intercourse but orgasm that may induce uterine contractions and, on occasion, premature birth *in those who have this tendency*. Therefore, if you have a tendency toward premature birth, then either intercourse or oral-genital contact should be without the attainment of orgasm.

There is only one note of caution, *which applies to pregnant women only*. The forceable blowing of air into the vagina can be absorbed by the many extra blood vessels in the pregnant uterus and result in air embolism with very serious consequences, even death on rare occasion.

I want to emphasize, however, that ordinary oral-genital contact is entirely permissible; it is only the forcing of air inwardly that should be avoided.

Dear Dr. Kaufman:

Until I reached the seventh month of pregnancy, sex relations with my husband were good, perhaps better than they had ever been. Now, I can't seem to enjoy sex in *any* position—we've tried all the recommended ones for the last third of pregnancy. My husband seems hurt by my lack of sexual desire, and I'm afraid he'll seek sexual satisfaction elsewhere.

Answer:

Occasionally a pregnant woman whose sex interest and response were heightened at one point develops a lack of desire and response (perhaps even an aversion) at another stage. This is usually a temporary reaction, almost always disappearing after delivery. Position during coitus may have to be modified as pregnancy advances; many women find it more comfortable astride the man or lying on the side. Apparently you have tried variations, including clitoral manipulations by hand or tongue, and still find diminished satisfaction.

It seems to me that you are emphasizing too much your own lack of desire. It would be more productive if you simply made sure your husband understands that you find him as appealing as ever and concentrate on pleasing him sexually.

Dear Dr. Kaufman:

I'm eight months' pregnant, and ever since about the fifth month, when I became very obviously pregnant, my husband seems to have very little desire for intercourse. He's not afraid it will hurt the baby, it's just that my big belly seems to turn him off. I still feel desire for him, and this—our first "sex problem"—is clouding an otherwise very happy pregnancy.

Answer:

Although many men are turned on by pregnancy (no contraception needed, etc.), some, alas, are turned off by a "big belly," as you state so perceptively. I am reminded of that delightful de Maupassant story about a man who has a passion for fat women, accepts one off the street for some lovemaking, only to find her unexpectedly in labor! Naturally the neighbors will not believe that the child is not his own, but for him the worst part is that afterward he finds her unattractively thin!

Obviously your situation is a temporary one and should not be viewed too seriously. There is no reason you cannot discuss your feelings frankly with your husband, and possibly try initiating sex play at unexpected times, which just might turn him on.

Dear Dr. Kaufman:

I'm less than two months' pregnant, and already my husband is treating me as though I'm made of glass. I don't mind his insisting on carrying packages, but when we make love he's so gentle that I'm not having orgasms and, though he *is*, I know sex isn't as satisfying for him either as it was when our lovemaking was more vigorous.

Answer:

Although your letter doesn't state it, I would guess that this is your first pregnancy and a very much desired one. The fact of the matter is that many first-time fathers-to-be experience this feeling of overprotectiveness together with an anxiety about not wishing to do any harm. The anxiety is not warranted, of course, but they can't help it. Neither can some men help feeling that a potential mother is a kind of "sacred vessel"—not a very sexy image!

With these points in mind, an understanding wife can better appreciate her husband's deepest, unexpressed feelings. Nevertheless, you can still discuss your own desires with him frankly, and even enlist the cooperation of your obstetrician, if needed, to point out that sexual relations during normal pregnancy cause no harm.

Dear Dr. Kaufman:

What advice do you have for pregnant women who smoke a lot?

Answer:

Quit.

Dear Dr. Kaufman:

How large is the actual embryo during the first few months of pregnancy?

Answer:

In the first month the embryo is approximately one quarter of an inch long, in the second month one inch long, in the third month four inches long, in the fourth month six inches long, in the fifth month ten inches long, and in the sixth month about twelve inches.

Dear Dr. Kaufman:

A friend of mine recently went to a clinic, where she was examined and treated by a nurse-midwife rather than a physician. Would this be considered proper care?

Answer:

To many people the mere mention of the word "midwife" conjures pictures of the Dark Ages or the backhills of Kentucky. Today, however, the type of "granny" midwife who practiced mainly in rural areas has been largely replaced by highly trained women who have degrees in nursing and many months of additional training in "midwifery." Such midwives are now relieving overworked doctors in delivery rooms throughout the country, and in clincs as well.

At most hospitals nurse-midwives tend only women who

are expected to deliver without complications. Of course, if there is any problem a doctor is called immediately. A midwife must, of course, know her limitations.

Two years ago the American College of Obstetricians and Gynecologists issued a statement enthusiastically endorsing the services of nurse-midwives.

Dear Dr. Kaufman:

I am considering having my child by "natural childbirth." How should I go about arranging it?

Answer:

So-called natural childbirth, sometimes called "educated" or "non-medicated" childbirth, was introduced as a concept by the English obstetrician, Grantly Dick-Read. He theorized that the main causes of discomfort during labor were fear and tense muscles. He advocated the elimination of fear through knowledge (classes, discussions, visual aids, not leaving the patient alone during labor, etc), and a program of relaxation exercises in preparation for labor. Ideally, the patient remains awake and a participant in her own labor and delivery, without the use or need for any drugs. However, Read recognized that not all patients are suitable candidates for natural childbirth (which some scientists feel is a form of self-hypnosis), and he stated that if the woman turns out to require pain relieving drugs or even deep anesthesia, she should not be denied such medication.

There is another form of natural childbirth, called the psychoprophylactic method, which is based on conditioned reflex. The concept, originally developed by the Russian, Pavlov, was popularized in France by Dr. Lamaze, and is referred to in this country as the Lamaze method. By repeated verbal instruction, an attempt is made to develop a conditioned reflex response toward the pains of labor. In fact, the term labor "pains" is never used, only "contractions." The woman is taught to counteract any discomfort by rehearsed relaxation exercises, and must actively participate in the entire labor and delivery process. While both the Read and Lamaze methods have things in common, it is the Lamaze method that seems to be the most popular in this country, possibly because it is considered by many to be somewhat more realistic in its approach.

Not all hospitals are geared for natural childbirth participants. Therefore it is important for any woman who is eager to try such a method to ask whether her obstetrician (and the hospitals with which he is associated) is able to provide this service. In fact, the woman should specifically choose an obstetrician who is familiar with the method she is interested in, and has used it frequently. As for formal instruction, the doctor may either hold his own "classes" or refer the patient (and her husband!) to courses given by nurses or other paraprofessionals, either in or out of hospital, according to the circumstances.

Just as not every hospital subscribes to natural childbirth, there are some women with low pain threshold who really prefer to be "out of it." There is no reason why she should force herself into a program of natural childbirth just because relatives or friends have been urging her. The best candidate for "natural" childbirth is the woman who does not wish to miss a minute of the whole process, and wants the exhilaration of actually seeing the birth of her own baby. Some hospitals not only encourage the husband's participation during the wife's labor, but permit him in the delivery room as well.

Of course, many women may be undecided. If so, I would advise them to prepare themselves by reading up on it, taking the classes, and discussing all the details with the obstetrician. There is much comfort in the realization that if the going gets rough, suitable medications will be given, and the woman should not have the slightest sense of guilt or of defeat. After all, it's the finished product that counts, and you'll have your baby for years to come no matter which "method" of childbirth you choose.

Dear Dr. Kaufman:

I am going to have a baby in eight months. I have heard that there are now several new pain killers available during childbirth. Could you tell me what they are and evaluate them. A friend of mine has told me how much pain she had having her baby, and I am frightened of having the same experience.

Answer:

Modern obstetrics has made much progress in the relief (and even elimination) of pain during childbirth and today no woman need suffer agonies. However, the methods I will describe are not really very "new" and have been in vogue for many years. The choices in each instance will necessarily be the ones with which the obstetrician is experienced and feels are best suited and safe for both mother and baby.

The most commonly used analgesic ("pain killer") is Demerol by injection, usually in combination with Scopolamine, an amnesic which clouds the memory. Occasionally a tranquilizer such as Sparine or Phenergan is added, which helps to deepen the total effect. The choice of drug or drugs to give, the exact amounts, and how often to repeat them are all decisions that the obstetrician must carefully weigh, since such drugs have at least the potential of making the baby sleepy too. Obviously every patient must have individual attention.

In addition to such analgesic pain killers, there are available a group of anesthetics to eliminate the pain of childbirth.

A "general" anesthetic (usually a gas by inhalation, but sometimes an intravenous solution) renders the mother completely unconscious for a relatively brief time. Even so, it may contribute to the sleepiness of the baby which, however, usually comes around quite quickly with careful handling right after delivery.

An alternate is the use of "conduction" or "regional" anesthesia, which acts locally and does not affect the baby. There are several types of conduction anesthesia. One is a low *spinal*, called "saddle block," which causes temporary paralysis from the waist down and stops labor as well. It is therefore used only when the patient is ready to deliver, and forceps (instrumental) delivery is generally necessary because of the absence of contractions. The mother's blood pressure must be carefully observed during spinal anesthesia, since there may be a temporary drop. In addition, about 6 per cent of such anesthetics are followed by rather severe headaches.

Another type of conduction anesthesia which produces less profound paralysis is an *epidural* "block," but there is still a good chance that the obstetrician will have to use forceps.

Still another type of conduction anesthesia is known as a *caudal*, which is given below the spinal canal so that the anesthetic simply bathes the nerve trunks as they make their exit. Since there is no motor paralysis and labor is not interfered with, a caudal can be started early, whenever labor has been well established. A plastic catheter, which substitutes for the needle, is then left in place, and additional amounts of anesthetic are injected as soon as the numbing effect begins to wear off. Caudal, then, serves as both an analgesic and an anesthetic, and is continued for as many hours as necessary until the delivery is over.

Since caudal anesthesia sounds so ideal, one may well ask why it isn't used routinely for everyone. There are several reasons. Since it is a technically difficult procedure, it requires special skill and much experience to make sure the needle is in exactly the right space. Once started, it then requires constant attendance by a physician or nurse to check the blood pressure, to decide when more anesthetic is needed, and so forth. Not all hospitals can supply such technical personnel at any given time. In addition, if it is given a bit too soon, or if contractions are not of a productive type, it may unduly prolong labor. And finally, some women are so constructed that their caudal canal is too narrow to enter altogether.

One other form of conduction anesthesia, which should not be overlooked, is a simple "local." This is given as soon as the baby is actually ready for delivery. The doctor injects one of the procaine-type drugs into suitable areas in and around the lower birth passage, which numbs the lower vagina as well as the area between the vagina and rectum. There is no interference with contractions, and with such local anesthesia the doctor can easily make (and then sew up) a cut to make more room for delivery.

Dear Dr. Kaufman:

A few weeks before the delivery of my last baby, I heard a rather loud clicking noise in my belly several times a day, usually when the baby moved. No one would believe me, and even my own doctor was skeptical. The baby was perfectly healthy when born. What could account for the noises? I know it was not just my imagination.

Answer:

Similar experiences have been reported from time to time in the medical literature. Such fetal clicks are probably due to the fact that the baby had hiccups! Although unusual, it appears to be an entirely normal event.

Dear Dr. Kaufman:

Can a woman who has two separate uteri give birth to two separate babies?

Answer:

Although it is extraordinarily rare, it has occurred. Two daughters were born to a young Cincinnati woman who had two separate and independent uteri, and the infants were really "litter mates" rather than twins, according to the medical report. She also had a partially divided vagina. The second pregnancy was thought to have begun two to six weeks after the first, and separate deliveries were planned. However, complications following the normal vaginal delivery of the first baby necessitated immediate delivery of the second one by Caesarean section.

Dear Dr. Kaufman:

People frequently talk about the "fine head of hair" in newborn infants. I was wondering when hair first makes its appearance in fetal life.

Answer:

Interestingly, the fetus's first meal is composed of its own hair! When the fetus is about 3½ months, a coat of fine hair sprouts from its skin. This lasts for another 3 months or so, when the hairs are shed into the surrounding amniotic fluid. Hairs are swallowed by the fetus and can be found undigested in the stool, which the child expels after birth. The fetal hairs that have remained on the skin are usually shed after birth, and are replaced by the delicate hair which is characteristic of the infant. At puberty, this delicate hair is again replaced, this time by the final "terminal" hair, which is regulated by the activity of the sex glands.

Dear Dr. Kaufman:

What is a phantom pregnancy?

Answer:

Phantom pregnancy (pseudocyesis) is believed to be caused by an intense desire for pregnancy. All the symptoms of pregnancy are present, including nausea, bloating of the abdomen, fullness of the breasts, and so on. However, the pregnancy test is negative, and examination reveals no enlargement of the uterus.

Dear Dr. Kaufman:

Is it possible to have menstrual periods while pregnant?

Answer:

On rare occasions a woman may have a menstrual period (as distinguished from abnormal bleeding) while pregnant. When this occurs, however, the bleeding is relatively scant and almost always ceases after one or two months.

Dear Dr. Kaufman:

Somewhere I read an incredible item, that some women

have a craving for things like dirt and starch when they are pregnant, in the belief that these things would be helpful. Is this just an old wives' tale?

Answer:

It is an old wives' tale that such things would be helpful, but I'm afraid it is true that there exists a common practice among some pregnant women to have a specific craving for clay, starch, baking soda, dirt, and other inedibles. It seems to be tied up with the belief that clay and starch prevent nausea, and keep the baby from being born with unsightly birthmarks or blemishes.

Dear Dr. Kaufman:

I understand that most states have passed laws requiring the screening of all newborn infants for a disease called phenylketonuria. What is this disease? I've never heard of it.

Answer:

Phenylketonuria is an inherited metabolic disorder associated with mental retardation. In spite of its low incidence, the disorder has aroused a good deal of interest because early nutritional management with foods low in phenylalanine can apparently prevent or lessen mental retardation.

Dear Dr. Kaufman:

How common is pregnancy in women over forty?

Answer:

Although approximately 150,000 live births occur each year to American women over the age of forty, in the vast majority of such cases it is in the early forties, becoming progressively more rare after 45.

Dear Dr. Kaufman:

Provided everything is normal, when is it all right to have sexual relations during pregnancy?

Answer:

At any time, from the beginning of conception to the time of labor. Incidentally, it is usually unnecessary to wait the customary six to eight weeks after delivery to permit intercourse again. It may be permitted as soon as it is comfortable, and that can be as early as four weeks, or even sooner in some cases.

Dear Dr. Kaufman:

What is the origin of the word *obstetrician?*

Answer:

From the Latin, meaning, "one who stands in front."

Dear Dr. Kaufman:

How long is the umbilical cord, and what is it composed of?

Answer:

The umbilical cord, a semi-transparent, jelly-like rope, averages 22 inches in length. It may normally be much shorter or longer. The cord contains three blood vessels—two arteries and one vein. Blood vessels run from the fetus through the cord, and then course through the placenta.

Answer:

The largest baby with authenticated birth weight was reported in 1933 in the *British Medical Journal.* The baby weighed 22 pounds, 2 ounces. The newborn was 35 inches long, and larger than the average child at one year. It was born dead. According to medical literature, no child has ever been born *alive* weighing more than 15½ pounds.

Dear Dr. Kaufman:

I fell on my stomach during my fourth month of pregnancy. There was no bleeding, but I'm still worried. What are the chances of harm to the baby?

Answer:

External trauma rarely harms the unborn child. If there is no vaginal bleeding within a few hours after the accident, one can assume that no damage has resulted to the pregnancy. Also, such accidents during pregnancy do not cause birthmarks or malformations.

Dear Dr. Kaufman:

Does the fetus swallow amniotic fluid? How much fluid is there at term?

Answer:

The fetus does swallow amniotic fluid and then excretes the fluid back into the amniotic sac in the form of fetal urine. At the end of nine months, there is usually about a quart of amniotic fluid. If the amount exceeds two quarts, the abnormal condition is called hydramnios.

Dear Dr. Kaufman:

I am 6½ months' pregnant, and when I lie down I feel quite certain that I can hear the baby's heart pulsating. This does not happen when I am in the standing position. Can you explain?

Answer:

What you are probably feeling is your own heartbeat, as transmitted by your aorta, the largest artery in your body. The pregnant uterus overlies it. If you time the beats, you will no doubt find that it is synchronous with your own pulse.

Dear Dr. Kaufman:

What is the purpose of the amniotic fluid surrounding the fetus?

Answer:

It is nature's shock absorber. A blow on the mother's abdomen merely jolts the fetus, and it floats away. The amniotic fluid also prevents the walls of the uterus from cramping the fetus and allows it unhampered growth and movement. The fluid is of constant temperature, a great insulator against the cold and heat.

Dear Dr. Kaufman:

I am 3 months' pregnant and even though I get about nine or ten hours of sleep at night, I'm still tired. Is this normal? Will taking more vitamins help?

Answer:

Overpowering sleepiness is a normal and common symptom during early pregnancy. Sleeping late or napping does not prevent this feeling, as you have already discovered, nor will taking more vitamins help.

Dear Dr. Kaufman:

About how much weight does a baby gain during the ninth (last) month of pregnancy?

Answer:

Approximately a half pound a week.

Dear Dr. Kaufman:

What is sickle cell disease, and how does it affect a pregnant woman?

Answer:

Sickle cell disease is an inherited, chronic hemolytic anemia characterized clinically by severe anemia, painful joints, and recurrent painful "crises." The disorder occurs almost exclusively in black persons. Many die within the first decade of life, and few survive to the age of forty.

Since there is no known cure, treatment is symptomatic. The pregnant woman with sickle cell disease seems especially susceptible to infection as well as other complications, maternal mortality being relatively high in these cases. Meticulous care during the prenatal period, labor, and postpartum period is essential.

Dear Dr. Kaufman:

What is hyaline membrane disease? I believe this was the disorder that the Kennedy infant died from.

Answer:

Hyaline membrane disease kills at least 20,000 newborns each year in the United States, most of them premature. There is a transparent coating or membrane (hyaline means glassy) that forms inside the lung air sacs, preventing oxygen from diffusing into the blood. There has been much progress in the detection and treatment of this disorder and the majority of babies with the disease recover completely.

Dear Dr. Kaufman:

I am 25 years old and am going to have my first baby in about four months. I am told at the clinic I go to that a cut will have to be made at the time of delivery, in order to make more room for the baby to come out. However, I wondered if it would be preferable, if possible, to avoid a cut and thus avoid a painful scar which might make sex uncomfortable later on.

Answer:

In an effort to avoid a cut in this area (with a first baby), the probabilities are that the muscle and connective tissue beneath the skin will be torn, and this may produce a relaxation of the muscles around the bladder and rectum, leading to less pleasurable sexual sensations for both partners. There is also a good possibility that the skin itself will tear anyway, requiring repair, and the scar will be much more ragged than one which is purposely made, as with the episiotomy planned. By the way, such a planned scar is rarely painful.

Dear Dr. Kaufman:

Is it true that a baby that is carried high usually turns out to be a boy?

Answer:

Babies are not carried "high" or "low." At certain stages of every pregnancy the baby's position may seem relatively higher or lower. Nor does the position bear any relationship to the baby's sex.

Dear Dr. Kaufman:

I was told at the clinic where I delivered that I had an "elective forceps" delivery. Why would the doctor "elect" to use forceps if the baby can be born without instruments?

Answer:

Elective forceps, also called "low" forceps, is a common form of delivery. It is true that in such cases the baby *could* be born without the use of forceps, but in many cases the doctor "elects" to use such "outlet" forceps for various reasons. One is to *slow* the birth so that the too rapid expulsion of the baby will not injure either the mother or infant. On other occasions it may be that the physical condition of the mother or baby is such that the obstetrician needs to hasten the birth. For example, there could be a change in the baby's heart rate, or in the position of the afterbirth. In general, first babies are more likely to require "elective" forceps than subsequent deliveries.

Dear Dr. Kaufman:

What is the mid-forceps procedure in childbirth?

Answer:

If the baby's head has come through the bony pelvic inlet but not past a certain spinous portion of the bony pelvis, a stronger pull is usually necessary, called "mid-forceps." Such procedures have decreased markedly in the past 10-15 years because of increased safety of Caesarean sections. Whether or not mid-forceps is used will depend upon the estimated size of the baby and the pelvis, the baby's position, the medical urgency to expedite the delivery, and the technical skill of the doctor.

Dear Dr. Kaufman:

I never gave much thought to postpartum blues until I experienced those dreaded feelings myself. Wow! I wonder if you could comment on the causes.

Answer:

Postpartum blues are believed to have both a psychological and physiological origin, with the emotional factors probably dominant. The new mother usually has the feeling of helplessness and confusion—like being trapped. A careful background history will probably reveal conflicts in assuming the motherhood role as well as conflicting advice from husband and family.

It is important to be aware that a *mild* degree of postpartum blues is present in the majority of normal women—such as crying episodes at some time during the first week or ten days after delivery. It is transient, benign, and apparently self-limiting. However, such a transient depression is unrelated to so-called postpartum psychosis, which is an uncommon but serious condition.

Dear Dr. Kaufman:

I would appreciate your comments on varicose veins during pregnancy.

Answer:

There is a general slowdown in the speed of blood flow during pregnancy. If a woman's veins tend to be weak, the extra pooled blood may cause them to bulge (varicose). Relief is usually obtained by elevating the legs and wearing elastic stockings. Varicose veins of the legs usually improve after childbirth.

Another kind of varicose vein that often troubles pregnant women is hemorrhoids—varicose veins of the rectum, which also improve a few weeks after delivery.

Dear Dr. Kaufman:

What exactly are stretch marks during pregnancy, and what causes them to appear in some women and not in others?

Answer:

Stretch marks are pinkish streaks in the skin. Such marks are not pigmentations but are rather due to decreased elasticity in the stretched skin over the growing uterus and often on the breasts too. Occasionally they appear on the thighs and buttocks as well.

Dear Dr. Kaufman:

I have read that twins occur about once in a hundred births. What about the incidence of triplets, quadruplets, etc.?

Answer:

Triplets occur once in about 10,000 births. Quadruplets have an incidence of once in 500,000. Quintuplets are actually too rare for any kind of accurate statistics. Their incidence has been estimated at about one in 15 to 20 million births. And sextuplets, which made headlines in 1973, are just too rare to evaluate.

Actually, 6 at once is not a record. There are a few cases of septuplets, all but one in Addis Ababa, and one reported case of octuplets in 1967 in Mexico City! (All 8 babies died within a day.)

Records are made to be broken, as the saying goes, and there is one reported case of nonuplets (9 babies), born in Australia in 1971; the mother had taken fertility drugs. Finally, the world's record is apparently the case reported from Rome, also in 1971. A woman is said to have miscarried 10 female and 5 male fetuses.

Dear Dr. Kaufman:

I was told that I was Rh negative, and although I don't have any children I would like to know as much as possible about Rh problems as they might affect me and any children I might have in the future.

Answer:

Back in 1939 it was discovered that a factor known as Rh was present in the blood of most people, designated as Rh positive, but *absent* in the blood of others (Rh negative). It was later realized that Rh disorders could occur only when an Rh negative mother was pregnant with an Rh positive baby who had inherited this blood from his Rh positive father. The Rh negative mother might produce antibodies to her unborn baby's Rh factor and these antibodies crossed the placenta and destroyed the baby's red blood cells. The result is "erythroblastosis fetalis" which, in its extreme form, could produce brain damage or a stillbirth.

One way of coping with the problem was an "exchange transfusion" after birth to exchange the baby's damaged blood with healthy blood. For some it was not possible to do this because the anemia was so great that it killed the fetus in the womb.

The next breakthrough came with the development of techniques to transfuse the baby *before* birth—intrauterine transfusions. Although sometimes successful, they are risky.

Now a new blood extract, a gamma globulin rich in Rh antibodies, enables doctors to protect each subsequent child merely by inoculating the mother within 3 days of birth or miscarriage. However, the vaccine is of no value in a woman already sensitized by previous childbirth, miscarriage, or abortion.

It should be emphasized that Rh disease rarely occurs with the first pregnancy, even when a mother is Rh negative and the baby is Rh positive. Subsequent pregnancies (without inoculation) may or may not be affected, according to whether there has been a build-up of maternal antibodies.

Dear Dr. Kaufman:

What is false labor? How can one tell it from real labor?

Answer:

False labor consists of uterine contractions which are usually irregular and cause no acute discomfort. It is common to have such contractions on and off during the last few weeks of pregnancy. False labor does not result in any progress in that there is no dilatation of the cervix.

In its early stages, true labor resembles false labor in that the contractions may also be irregular and relatively painless. However, in true labor the pattern soon changes in that the contractions become more regular, come at progressively shorter intervals, and become increasingly uncomfortable as the womb begins to dilate.

Dear Dr. Kaufman:

What is the basis for the oft-quoted saying that a baby born in the seventh month of pregnancy has a better chance for survival than one born in the eighth month?

Answer:

The myth probably got started because in certain toxic conditions, the sooner the baby got "out' the better. But prematurity poses great dangers and, in general, the longer the period of gestation, the better.

Dear Dr. Kaufman:

Why was I referred to as an "elderly primipara" just because I am 36? That doesn't sound too old to me.

Answer:

In obstetrical jargon, any woman who is pregnant for the first time after age 35 is classified under the unflattering heading of "elderly." The reason is that labor is usually longer, and the childbearing span of women at 35 is more than two-thirds over. Maternal and fetal risks are also somewhat higher in older women.

Dear Dr. Kaufman:

I hear a lot about "advances" in modern obstetrics and wondered if you could elaborate on some of these.

Answer:

Electronic monitoring of the fetal heart is certainly one significant advance.

There are also several tests which help to give the "high risk" baby a better chance. One is called the lecithin-sphingomyelin (L-S) ratio, which tests the amniotic fluid for certain fatty substances that reflect fetal lung maturity. Sometimes there are plans to deliver a baby early because of conditions such as previous Caesarean section, Rh sensitization, maternal diabetes, or toxemia. Since the majority of neonatal deaths are due to respiratory problems, such assessment of fetal lung maturity is a valuable clue as to whether early delivery can be carried out with relative safety.

Another test is the estriol level obtained from the maternal urine, collected over a 24-hour span, which reflects fetal-placental function. A low or falling level can be an indication that the fetus is in danger and helps the obstetrician decide whether to deliver the baby earlier than planned.

THREE

Complications of Pregnancy

Dear Dr. Kaufman:

I have had three pregnancies all ending in miscarriages in the early weeks. Is there any point in trying again?

Answer:

Three or more miscarriages constitute a condition known as "habitual abortion," and should be thoroughly investigated before any further attempts are made to conceive.

Such investigations could include an x-ray of your uterus to see if it is misshapen, genetic chromosome studies, and perhaps a culture to determine if there are present such elusive virus-like organisms as T. Mycoplasma, which recently have been implicated in some cases of repeated miscarriages.

Dear Dr. Kaufman:

I knew a young woman who recently almost died from a tubal pregnancy, and I am curious to learn about the symptoms and warning signs. The woman did not even know that she was pregnant. Do periods come regularly, late, or not at all?

Answer:

A tubal (ectopic) pregnancy is one that get trapped in one of the Fallopian tubes. Often the fertilized egg just stops growing, and there are very few symptoms and no unusual consequences. However, if the embryo continues to develop, it may burst through the tube, causing internal hemorrhage. This requires immediate surgery.

There may or may not be a missed period. In fact, the egg may be fertilized, get caught in the tube, and burst through it even before a single period is missed! This is one reason that an ectopic pregnancy often goes unsuspected until the onset of sudden pain or other symptoms. The treatment of a tubal pregnancy is by surgical removal as soon as the diagnosis is definitely made. Fatalities are rare.

Although over 90 per cent of ectopic pregnancies occur in the Fallopian tube, they can be found in other sites. An *abdominal* pregnancy is the result of the embryo's breaking out of the tube and attaching itself to neighboring organs such as the intestine or the abdominal lining. It may continue to develop and even approach full term! However, the number of babies who survive an abdominal pregnancy is extremely small. If the abdominal pregnancy is not diagnosed as such, there is no way for the fetus to enter the birth canal and it will die unless delivered surgically.

Ectopic pregnancies can occur, very rarely, in two other sites. If an egg cell cannot escape from the ovary and is fertilized there, an embryo can develop there, called an *ovarian* pregnancy. Finally, if a fertilized egg travels into the uterus and keeps going, it is possible for it to be embedded in the lining of the cervix, which is called a *cervical* pregnancy.

Cervical pregnancies have even been reported in women who have had partial hysterectomies, where the cervix was not removed!

Dear Dr. Kaufman:

My last pregnancy ended in a miscarriage at nine weeks, but the doctor said there was no fetus—just some grape-like clusters. How is this explained?

Answer:

You have described a typical "mole," which is an abnormality in the development of embryonic tissue. No real fetus forms, and miscarriage is inevitable.

Dear Dr. Kaufman:

I am a clinic patient and have not gotten a very clear answer to a problem which worries me. I miscarried what the doctors called a "hydatid mole" almost a year ago. Ever since, I have had numerous blood tests, urine tests, and even x-rays. The doctors tell me everything is all right, but why all these tests if that is so?

Answer:

Every mole has a small potential of becoming malignant. Even after the mole is extruded, there may be fragments within the uterus that can behave in a malignant fashion, even spreading to other organs such as the chest. That is why various tests are done, to determine whether there is any persistent or rising level of "pregnancy hormone," which would alert the doctor to such a possibility, and call for special treatment.

Dear Dr. Kaufman:

I read somewhere that an ordinary pregnancy can turn into a cancer. How is this possible?

Answer:

There is a rare condition produced by pregnancy which is called a choriocarcinoma. It is a definite cancer and usually arises during pregnancy from an abnormally developing cell structure that is called a mole (grape-like cluster). In 90-95 per cent of such cases, moles are benign, but in the remainder they can turn into an invasive cancer.

It is even more rare for a choriocarcinoma to follow a normal, full-term delivery, but this can occur.

It is absolutely essential to follow up and monitor every mole with hormone levels since this is the earliest barometer of a possibly developing cancer. Even if choriocarcinoma does develop, highly effective chemotherapy is available. If the diagnosis is made early enough, a complete cure may be expected in over 90 per cent of the cases.

Dear Dr. Kaufman:

I am 32 years old and have been trying to become pregnant for the past few months. My periods are fairly regular, every 28 or 29 days. However, my last period came five days late and was heavier than usual. Was this a miscarriage?

Answer:

The history you give strongly suggests an early miscarriage, but it is not possible to prove it. The fact that you were a few days late is significant in view of your previously regular cycles, though a delayed ovulation would result in a similarly delayed menstrual period. However, the heavier bleeding could represent an early miscarriage. Interestingly, tissue studies have shown that miscarriages can occur even earlier—without even missing a period. These miscarriages have been described as "silent abortions." I must emphasize, however, that such a diagnosis cannot be made without the specific evidence of microscopie studies of tissue obtained from, or expelled from, the uterus.

Dear Dr. Kaufman:

My doctor said I have a threatened miscarriage. I am eight weeks pregnant. My only symptoms are slight staining and a little cramping. He prescribed only bedrest, but I was wondering if there is anything else that can be done to save this pregnancy; I want the baby very much.

Answer:

Treatment of threatened miscarriage is variable, ranging from no therapy at all to bedrest, sedation, reassurance, hormonal therapy, and even psychotherapy, depending upon the preferences of the particular physician. The point is that equally good (or poor) results have been claimed by almost every form of therapy advocated, including doing nothing at all.

Sometimes progesterone deficiency is thought to play a role. In such cases, giving progesterone would, at least theoretically, be of help; it is often given, however, without really being sure whether such deficiency exists.

The use of estrogen, in particular diethylstilbestrol, is not considered safe therapy, since in recent years there have been some cases of vaginal or cervical cancer in female offspring of mothers who were given large amounts of this drug during early pregnancy.

Obviously all treatment will fail if the embryonic tissue is defective, a not infrequent occurrence. One should also bear in mind that if a woman who is treated with a particular medication does carry to term, it does not prove that the medication was the determining factor, though it would probably be given the credit.

Dear Dr. Kaufman:

Is there any relationship between the amount of bleeding in threatened miscarriage and the chances of holding the baby?

Answer:

Yes. The chances of holding the baby are better if the bleeding is light and stops within a week.

Dear Dr. Kaufman:

If a woman has had two consecutive miscarriages, what are her future chances of carrying to term?

Answer:

Various studies have indicated that between 50 and 80 percent of patients who have had two miscarriages continued their next pregnancy to term.

Dear Dr. Kaufman:

I had an uncomplicated early abortion about 4 years ago and now, for the last two years, I have been unable to conceive. Naturally I am worried that the abortion may have harmed my fertility somehow. What are the chances of this being the problem?

Answer:

Although it is a possibility, there are so many other factors that may impede fertility that only a complete investigation can disclose the true cause or causes for your present problem. There is a natural tendency to feel guilt, especially about a previous abortion; but keep in mind that many women have had multiple abortions without necessarily interfering with their fertility.

Dear Dr. Kaufman:

Do uterine fibroids interfere with fertility? If a woman with fibroids is already pregnant, is there a greater chance of miscarriage? If at term, is labor or delivery interfered with?

Answer:

Small fibroids do not often interfere with fertility, though they certainly don't help it either. If a woman with fibroids desires children, it is important to exclude other possible causes of infertility in both partners.

Once pregnancy has taken place, there are two ways in which a woman with fibroids may have a greater tendency to miscarry. If fibroids are large, there may be encroachment upon the uterine cavity and insufficient expansion for the fetus. Even if small, a fibroid that projects into the uterine cavity is often responsible for spontaneous miscarriage.

During more advanced pregnancy, fibroids may increase markedly in size and give rise to much pain from degeneration. During labor, fibroids may induce an abnormal fetal position and occasionally affect uterine contractions. However, actual mechanical obstruction from fibroids is relatively rare, since fibroids generally develop high in the uterus. Immediately after delivery, the uterus may not contract properly due to fibroids, with resulting increased bleeding. Within a few weeks after childbirth, fibroids generally shrink in size.

Dear Dr. Kaufman:

I have a theory about a cause of premature births and wonder what you think of it. You know how a nursing infant stimulates the mother's uterus to contract? Well, if a woman is pregnant and her husband keeps fondling her breasts during sex relations, it seems to me that her uterus would be stimulated to contract in the same way. You know what I mean?

Answer:

I do know what you mean, but I can't agree. If that were the case, the incidence of prematurity would be almost 100 per cent! Besides, uterine responsiveness to breast suckling after delivery is quite different than before.

FOUR

Why Can't I Get Pregnant?

Dear Dr. Kaufman:

In your various writings on infertility, I have noticed that you often speak of infertility studies as "medical sleuthing." Do you really liken this to detective work?

Answer:

Yes. In formal detective stories doctors make excellent detectives because, occupationally, they enjoy drawing inferences. Diagnosis, after all, is very much like detective work.

Sherlock Holmes was, in fact, created by a physician, Arthur Conan Doyle. Holmes himself was supposedly modeled after Doyle's surgical professor, Dr. Joseph Bell. And it is the good physician Dr. Watson, who recounts most of the episodes. Although Doyle's super sleuth was not himself a physician, he relied heavily on Dr. Watson's help and companionship in most of his cases.

Dear Dr. Kaufman:

I have read that a woman produces about 400 or 500 ova in a lifetime. About how many of these are of good fertilizable quality?

Answer:

A female child's ovaries start out with some 4 million potential ova and it is true that only about 400 or 500 of these are ever involved in ovulation. All the rest degenerate, or are resorbed within the ovaries.

Of eggs that actually come into contact with sperm, the great majority don't make it through early cleavage stages or during implantation. Others are lost by absorption or by spontaneous abortion. Only about a third result in live births, including one per cent born with congenital abnormalities. Thus, only about a third of fertilized eggs are apparently of "good quality."

Dear Dr. Kaufman:

How much of the total ejaculate that a male produces is actually sperm?

Answer:

Sperm comprise only about 0.1% of the total ejaculate. And it is the first portion of the ejaculate that contains most of them.

Dear Dr. Kaufman:

Does sperm quality change as a man gets older?

Answer:

In men who remain sexually active, the sperm count will not change if the semen quality was initially good. However, whenever sexual activity declines appreciably, the sperm's capacity for movement, or "motility," is usually diminished. In such instances there is usually no appreciable effect upon the sperm count, which may actually show a slight increase due to longer periods of abstinence.

Dear Dr. Kaufman:

How comparable are sperm and egg cells?

Answer:

Sperm are expendable; they are produced by the billions. Eggs are very precious; only about twelve or thirteen are produced each year. Think about that!

Dear Dr. Kaufman:

I understand that the "basal" body temperature record is a common test to show whether a woman ovulates. When was this correlation first observed as a medical phenomenon?

Answer:

Van De Velde showed that the basal temperature graph was associated with ovulation in 1904. Today, the procedure continues to be one of the simplest and most popular means of ovulation detection. Such waking temperatures can be taken by mouth, which is the preferred way. Normally, the record shows a typical two-plateau pattern during an ovulatory cycle. The second, higher level is associated with an increased production of progesterone from the ovaries.

It should be emphasized that the basal temperature record does not *predict* the day of ovulation, but rather provides evidence that ovulation has already taken place, 2-3 days after it occurs.

Dear Dr. Kaufman:

I was wondering how the criteria for "normal" sperm was established, inasmuch as there would appear to be no reason for normal, fertile men to have their sperm analyzed.

Answer:

This is a subject about which I can speak first-hand, since my first medical article was called "What is a Normal Semen?" and appeared in the *Journal of Human Fertility* (March, 1946). In trying to establish a "norm," I analyzed voluntarily given specimens from men whose wives were pregnant and attending the prenatal clinic at the hospital where I was resident in gynecology.

It was delicate work, often embarrassing, since I had to obtain sperm from men who could see no particular reason to part with it. I managed to persuade them that it was somehow important for a better understanding and care of their wives. The data, together with similar studies by others, did help to clarify the question of what was "normal."

Dear Dr. Kaufman:

How important is timing of intercourse when there is an infertility problem? We have been trying to have a baby for almost two years, and wonder whether we just haven't picked the right time, though we have relations rather frequently.

Answer:

Incorrect timing is definitely not a cause of long-standing infertility and is obviously not the cause of your problem. Over a span of two years, you have surely had intercourse on every "conceivable" day of the cycle many times over. Other factors are undoubtedly playing a role, and should be properly investigated.

Dear Dr. Kaufman:

We are eager to have a baby. Our doctor advised us to have intercourse every other night, but another doctor suggested we have relations every night during my fertile time. My husband is exhausted! Do you think such advice is helpful?

Answer:

On the contrary, I must say frankly that such advice, no matter how well meaning, can be needlessly upsetting. In my opinion, regimenting sex serves no useful purpose whatsoever. And the fact that it's "doctor's orders" doesn't make it any better.

An infertile marriage is frustrating enough without adding instructions which can make a couple's sex life equally frustrating. If you normally have sex relations two or three times a week, that's good enough and one should look for other causes to explain the infertility problem. The guide for sex should not be a calendar or temperature graph, but desire alone.

Dear Dr. Kaufman:

I have been trying to become pregnant for over a year, and the thought occurred to me that maybe we were trying too hard. Is it possible that sperm are weakened by too frequent intercourse (five or six times a week)?

Answer:

Frequent ejaculations can lower the sperm count and total volume somewhat, but there is essentially no effect on the most important aspect of sperm quality, which is their capacity for movement. Since you have been trying for over a year, it would be advisable to consult a physician. In all probability, your frequency of intercourse is not a cause of your problem. In fact, at all levels of fertility, the greater the frequency of intercourse, the greater the chances of conception since there is more exposure and the sperm capacity for movement is, if anything, improved. No doubt other factors will be found to play a role in your infertility problem.

Dear Dr. Kaufman:

What are the common causes of infertility in women? How are these causes detected?

Answer:

The ovaries may not be producing egg cells, or the eggs may lack sufficient vitality due to improper functioning of the pituitary, thyroid, or other glands. Keeping a basal (waking) temperature graph may provide an early clue. In addition, an "egg test" or endometrial biopsy, which is the examination of a bit of uterine lining taken at a certain time of the cycle, reflects the quality of the egg. There are also tests for the function of the various glands concerned with menstruation and ovulation.

The tubes may be narrowed or closed, making it impossible for an egg to enter. The Rubin test, or tubal insufflation, consists of passing carbon dioxide gas slowly through the tubes to see if the tubes are open without undue pressure being required. Normally there is shoulder pain on sitting up right after the test, indicating that gas has passed through the tubes. Another way of examining the tubes is by hysterosalpingography, which is an x-ray of the inside of the uterus and tubes, after instilling a special dye. Any blockage of the narrow tubal passage is shown by a stoppage of dye at that point. Still another, and more comprehensive way of evaluating the tubes is by endoscopy, a minor operative procedure wherein a special visualizing instrument is inserted either through the vagina (culdoscopy) or the abdomen (laparoscopy).

Another common cause of infertility is the inability of normal sperm to gain entry in sufficient numbers into the womb. The failure to ascend through the cervical canal is detected by the postcoital test. This test, done at midcycle when the cervical secretions are most hospitable, consists of taking secretions from various levels of the cervical canal to see if there are sufficient numbers of actively motile sperm present. The failure of normal sperm to gain a good "beachhead" in the cervix may be due to a chronic inflammation in that region or to glandular disturbance that results in hostile secretions.

Infertility in women is not only the inability to conceive, but may take the form of inability to "hold" a pregnancy after conception. The occurrence of multiple miscarriages is always a frustrating problem. A meticulous investigation is needed, including a search for hormonal deficiencies, anatomic defects, constitutional or nutritional factors, and emotional factors.

Dear Dr. Kaufman:

Having read your book on infertility, I know that you do not favor sex on schedule. That's probably good advice for the average couple, but what would you say of my own case, where my husband is away a lot? Since we want to have a baby, wouldn't you say that his homecoming should be specifically timed to the day or days when I am most fertile?

Answer:

It would make sense in your particular case, which is an exception.

In this regard, I am reminded of an incident years ago, about an infertility patient whose husband was a traveling salesman, away from home more often than not. This patient had moved to Canada and had sent me her basal temperature graph to look over in advance of a person-to-person phone call that she would make regarding further advice on coital "timing." When my secretary buzzed me that the awaited call from Canada was on the line, I was all prepared with the temperature graph before me, lifted the receiver and said, "Hi! When was the last time you had intercourse?" "I *beg* your pardon!" came the indignant voice of the long distance operator, who had not yet made the connection.

Dear Dr. Kaufman:

I recently had an after-intercourse test for investigation of an infertility problem, and had to rush to the doctor's office for examination as soon as possible after I had relations. Yet another doctor, in doing the same test, said it didn't matter—I could arrive for examination several hours later. Because of these conflicting instructions, I am confused.

Answer:

Years ago it was the general feeling that the post-coital test had to be done as soon as possible after intercourse. However, various research studies have shown that it is really not necessary to rush, and that the findings many hours later are in some ways even more revealing. I personally do not impose any time limit for my patients who undergo this test. In fact, it is not uncommon for a husband to rebel against "performing" on request in the morning, and I have accepted results based on more relaxed coitus even the night before.

Dear Dr. Kaufman:

We have an infertility problem. My husband has had two sperm counts, done by the same laboratory, a week apart. One was 30 million and the other was 110 million. How do you account for the difference?

Answer:

Although there are normal variations in sperm counts from week to week and from day to day, it is difficult to account for the wide variation you mention, assuming your husband remained in good health. Many laboratories are not equipped to do accurate sperm analyses; a trained urologist or gynecologist could probably clarify not only your husband's sperm count but other important aspects of the semen such as the motility and anatomic abnormalities.

Dear Dr. Kaufman:

My husband was told that his sperm count and motility were subnormal, though his health is excellent. Could there be a physical cause for this that is not obvious?

Answer:

He might have a varicocele (varicose veins in the scrotum), which is sometimes associated with the type of sperm abnormality you describe. If so, surgical correction may improve the picture. A urologist should evaluate his condition.

Sometimes a glandular disturbance plays a role, and this can usually be corrected. However, often there is no apparent cause for such sperm deficiency, and it is simply called "congenital."

Dear Dr. Kaufman:

I am 33 years old and we have three children. About six months ago my husband got sick with mumps, and it affected his testicles. Can I safely give up contraception now? I understand that mumps involving the testicles causes sterility in the male.

Answer:

Testicular mumps usually, *but not always,* leads to male sterility. I know of one case where the husband had a very severe mumps orchitis (testicular inflammation) and assumed he was sterile. His wife conceived a few months later.

Your husband's seminal fluid should be tested to see if it still contains sperm. That way, you would not be guessing.

Dear Dr. Kaufman:

I am particularly interested in so-called psychogenic infertility: that is, where there is no physical cause, but there is infertility from emotional causes. My question is, how can the emotions actually prevent fertilization? If it *is* possible, then how is it that rape victims so often become pregnant, when you would expect whatever mechanism is at work in psychogenic infertility to prevent conception in situations like that?

Answer:

Psychogenic infertility is indeed a most interesting phenomenon and rather poorly understood. However, it is not that the woman can "will" that there be no conception, but rather, the emotional factors are mediated through physical or physiological pathways to prevent conception. For example, I recall one patient who claimed she very much wanted to have a baby. At the same time, however, she complained of almost constant vaginal spotting, and refused to have intercourse because of this. It was found that her staining was due to the fact that no egg was being produced, with resultant fluctuating estrogen levels producing the spotting. It was only after extensive counseling and questioning that it became apparent that she actually was afraid of pregnancy because she was sure her marriage would not last. Her vaginal bleeding gave her a respectable excuse for avoiding intercourse, while inhibition of ovulation protected her against pregnancy.

Rape situations are quite different in that there is no prior deep-seated problem that operates to prevent conception through physical or physiological mechanisms. The victim is caught by surprise and, in fact, there is some evidence (though controversial) that, contrary to the victim's will, ovulation may actually be triggered by the stress situation, thus facilitating conception.

Dear Dr. Kaufman:

I have been told that my tubes are closed. Where does the egg go each month if it cannot get into the tube?

Answer:

It falls by the wayside. Even if the tubes are open, it does not mean that the extruded egg will necessarily fall into one of them. If it doesn't make it, the egg (which is really almost microscopic in size) simply drops into the abdominal cavity and is absorbed. If it does get into the tube and is not fertilized, it will find its way into the womb and will then be cast off during the next menstrual period.

Dear Dr. Kaufman:

Can a woman menstruate without ovulating? Can she ovulate without menstruating? Are regular periods a sign of good fertility?

Answer:

These are frequently asked questions. A woman can menstruate without ovulating. In such cases, periods are usually, but not always, irregular.

The second question is a little more tricky. A woman who ovulates will always menstruate about two weeks later unless pregnancy intervenes. The only other exception is the rare instance where the endometrium (uterine lining) has been so destroyed by surgery or disease that it is completely unresponsive.

From the fertility standpoint, one can say that a woman whose periods are normal and regular probably ovulates, while a woman with grossly irregular cycles is at best ovulating erratically, if at all.

Dear Dr. Kaufman:

A friend of mine was told she had "hard-shelled ovaries" and would need an operation to correct the condition. She has been unable to become pregnant for almost four years. Could you explain what this condition is?

Answer:

So-called hard-shelled ovaries are capable of being stimulated by the woman's own pituitary gland, but the maturing eggs cannot be extruded because of a thick, hard capsule covering the ovaries. A lot of unextruded eggs collect under such a capsule, often giving the ovary a characteristic "polycystic" appearance, also known in some instances as the Stein-Leventhal syndrome. The best way to be sure of the diagnosis is by direct visualization.

Among the common treatments for such ovaries are cortisone by-products and the fertility pill, clomiphene. However, if there is no response after several months of such treatment in high dosage (and combined with other hormonal preparations), then an operation may be considered as a final resort. In this procedure, "wedges" are removed from both ovaries and all remaining cysts obliterated by puncturing. Exactly why this operation should result in the resumption of ovulation and consequent pregnancy in a substantial percentage of cases is not clear.

Dear Dr. Kaufman:

How does a woman know for sure that she is ovulating?

Answer:

The only absolutely sure sign that ovulation has definitely occurred is the presence of pregnancy! However, there are a number of presumptive symptoms, signs and tests that leave little room for doubt. The temperature graph is a strong presumptive sign of ovulation, when it has the typical biphasic pattern. Some women have mid-month pain, about fourteen days before the onset of the next period. It is called "ovulation pain" since it can often be correlated with other signs of ovulation, such as slight staining at the time, or an increased slippery discharge for a few days. The presence of premenstrual tension or painful periods constitute additional presumptive signs that ovulation has occurred. (This does not mean that women with painless periods don't ovulate!).

In addition, there are various hormonal tests of a complex nature which would go along with ovulation, as well as the finding of a "secretory" type of uterine lining on biopsy.

Dear Dr. Kaufman:

I read something about a "fern test" for cervical mucus. What is this test used for?

Answer:

A characteristic of cervical mucus in women who ovulate is the appearance—and disappearance—of a fern-leaf-like pattern when dried cervical mucus is viewed under a microscope. Ferning begins early in the cycle, reaching maximum patterns at ovulation time, then gradually disappears. It is caused indirectly by estrogen stimulation, but actually by the presence of salt in the mucus. For that reason, any salt solution (even a drop of ink) will show the same microscopic picture. The fern test has limitations, since the presence of cervical infection or staining may interfere with the test.

Dear Dr. Kaufman:

What is the so-called "fertility pill" I keep hearing about? Is this hormone associated with quadruplets and quintuplets?

Answer:

Contrary to popular belief, the so-called fertility pill (clomiphene citrate) is *not* a hormone at all, but is a synthetic chemical that is capable of stimulating the ovaries to produce ova in many instances. The mechanism of action is not completely understood, and the doctor must make an individual judgment as to when to use it.

Although there is a somewhat greater than average chance of twins with the fertility pill (clomiphene), this is *not* the drug that has been so notoriously publicized in connection with quadruplets and quintuplets. That drug is Pergonal, an injectable hormonal preparation.

Dear Dr. Kaufman:

Could you discuss the fertility drug that has resulted in so many highly publicized instances of multiple pregnancies?

Answer:

You are probably referring to the hormonal preparation, Pergonal, which has an interesting background. The knowledge that postmenopausal women have a high level of pituitary secretion led to the successful isolation of a follicle-stimulating hormone to help younger, infertile women who lack enough of this pituitary substance and consequently do not ovulate. Extracted from the urine of postmenopausal women, Pergonal is therefore known also as human menopausal gonadotropin (HMG). Pergonal alone will not usually induce ovulation, but it has been found that the addition of human chorionic gonadotropin (HCG), easily obtained from the urine of pregnant women, constitutes one of the most potent ovulation stimulants known. Although the occurrence of multiple pregnancies associated with Pergonal is well known, such possibilities can be minimized by careful dosage regulation and frequent monitoring for signs of overstimulation.

Dear Dr. Kaufman:

When was artificial insemination first used?

Answer:

The first reported instance of artificial insemination was thought to be in the fourteenth century, and had a rather destructive objective. An Arabic story dating around 1312 recounts how warring tribes injected their enemies' thoroughbred mares with semen from inferior stallions. Actually an even earlier report can be said to be a Talmudic document which antedates the Arabic tale by about 1100 years, and is concerned with a hypothetical discussion of a woman who had become unknowingly inseminated by semen previously deposited in the bath water in which she bathed. However, the report was academic and did not refer to *intentional* donor insemination.

If we first consider artificial insemination with the *husband's* sperm, the first English reference tells of the English surgeon, John Hunter, who artificially impregnated the wife of a London linen merchant. A normal pregnancy and delivery followed. In 1866 the noted American gynecologist J. Marion Sims reported that he had performed 55 artificial inseminations on six women which resulted in the first American test tube baby. To my knowledge, none of the publications prior to 1900 mentioned the use of donor semen.

In the United States, the pioneer of *donor* insemination was the late Dr. Robert L. Dickinson, who began using this procedure in secrecy during the 1890's. To this man belongs the greatest share of the credit for the increasing practice and acceptance of this therapeutic procedure. However, it should also be mentioned that for many decades, animal husbandry had developed artificial insemination into a constructive science for the breeding and improvement of the stock.

Dear Dr. Kaufman:

Is artificial donor insemination widely used today?

Answer:

Yes. Therapeutic (a better term) donor insemination has resulted in thousands of babies born to be loved in thousands of homes made happier. The number of "repeat" cases attests to the popularity of the procedure and the satisfactions gained.

Both husband and wife must want this procedure, and the marriage must have good stability before the procedure can be seriously considered by the conscientious physician.

Dear Dr. Kaufman:

I have often wondered whether couples who have a child by donor insemination really feel the same as those who have one of their own. With your wide experience along those lines, I'm sure you are in a good position to compare.

Answer:

Because of the infertility problem, donor babies are often *more* appreciated than those which are conceived and born at will. Exactly how the parents feel is well depicted by a letter I received from a patient who became pregnant by donor insemination, had her baby in her home state, and sent me a photo of her newborn with the following note:

"At least a million of these you must have seen, both in the flesh and in photos, but I know you'll recognize the unparalleled beauty of this one. I recall your examining me when I was eight weeks' pregnant and quite disbelieving, and your saying, 'You have a beautiful baby in there.'

"The whole of my pregnancy was wonderfully uneventful, and

the delivery (which was 2 days before your predicted date) as smooth and happy as possible. Jim was with me the entire time (he's responsible for this picture and about 30 others, several double-exposed amidst the excitement). Being unwilling to miss a minute of something we wanted so much for so long, I had no anesthesia so we both experienced the whole birth totally aware. And it was, as you well know, miraculous. . . .

Fondly,"

Dear Dr. Kaufman:

What can be done for infertility if the only thing wrong is some weakness in the sperm? At the clinic I go to, they told me my husband's sperm had only fair motility and the numbers were less than average. Everything else seemed to check out all right.

Answer:

The first thing to determine is whether there is anything in his own makeup that might be causing subnormal sperm. Sometimes a thyroid or other hormonal deficiency can have such an effect, and sometimes a varicocele (varicose veins of the scrotum) can contribute to poor sperm motility.

If there are no correctible factors, and if all of your own tests are completely normal, then some specialists have used a method called therapeutic husband insemination. A few drops from the first (best) portion of the fresh ejeculate, collected in a sterile container, are instilled high in the cervical canal, or even into the uterine cavity directly. This gives the sperm a valuable "head start," so to speak, when their own power of motion is relatively weak.

Dear Dr. Kaufman:

Can a woman have vaginal bleeding from emotional causes? How can you be sure?

Answer:

A woman can indeed bleed for emotional reasons, and one usually cannot be certain this is the case at the time it's happening unless it's like a startling case I had not long ago.

This was a 39-year-old woman who wanted desperately to have a baby, and she was getting intrauterine inseminations with her husband's (weak) sperm to give a needed "boost." She became pregnant but unfortunately miscarried two months later. We resumed inseminations and for several months nothing happened. One day she called to say she was bleeding unexpectedly and heavily. Examination disclosed no physical cause. The bleeding continued unabated until she had a startling revelation during the night that these were the "bloody tears of a disappointed uterus" and that this was the month she *would* have had her baby if she had not miscarried! At first I brushed this explanation aside, calling her attention to the fact that the "bloody tears" expression was not original and was even quoted in one of my books. She assured me she had never heard it before, and had not read my book. When she saw that I was still skeptical she added the zinger that her bleeding stopped as soon as she awakened from her dream as mysteriously as it had started!

Dear Dr. Kaufman:

I conceived easily three years ago, but have been unable to become pregnant since then. What could be wrong?

Answer:

The fact that pregnancy took place easily in the past is

certainly a good sign of fertility. Obviously something has changed since then. One frequent cause is that the Fallopian tubes, which normally receive the egg each month, become narrowed or blocked, due to an irritative reaction from previous delivery. There are tests to determine if this is so, as well as remedies.

Another cause is that the sperm, though normal, are unable to reach the egg due to unreceptive secretions in the cervix. This can be due either to a low-grade inflammation or a hormonal imbalance.

Whether or not an egg is being produced each cycle also needs investigation. This includes hormonal studies, because several glands affect fertility.

Dear Dr. Kaufman:

I have read somewhere that withdrawal can help infertile couples conceive a child. Isn't that paradoxical, since withdrawal is a method of contraception?

Answer:

The type of withdrawal that you have heard about is not withdrawal after ejaculation, but withdrawal after the *first portion* of the ejaculate has been emitted. This is based on the principle that the majority of sperm, and also the best ones, are contained in the first portion of the ejaculate. If the sperm happen to be below average in fertility, this method could, in effect, expose the woman to a superior (more concentrated) portion of seminal fluid and thus help in her efforts to conceive.

Dear Dr. Kaufman:

I am 37 years old and have fibroids. I am told that there are three, each about the size of a walnut. I am recently married and wonder if it is possible to conceive with this condition and if this could cause problems during pregnancy or at birth.

Answer:

Whether or not fibroids (benign fibromuscular growths of the womb) interfere with fertility depends more on their exact location than upon their size. Those on the surface of the womb are much less likely to interfere with conception than those that may press into the cavity of the uterus. The latter may not only hinder fertility—they may sometimes cause a miscarriage. Fortunately, they are much less common than surface fibroids.

Because fertility also diminishes as a woman gets older, you would be well advised not to wait too long before starting your family.

Dear Dr. Kaufman:

I have read somewhere that sexual intercourse itself cannot induce ovulation in women. Is this true?

Answer:

On the contrary, there is evidence for coitus-induced ovulation in human females. The documentation has to do with certain stress situations. For example, they include conceptions resulting from rape; conceptions resulting from limited exposure (as when the husband is away for long periods of time); and also during the stress of extramarital affairs.

The opposite reaction may also occur; that is, absence of periods due to stress. This may be from simple anxiety, such as fear of becoming pregnant, or from emtional trauma as widely seen during wartime.

Dear Dr. Kaufman:

I have a problem. I would like to get pregnant and do need some vaginal lubrication, but I am afraid that whatever lubrication I use will interfere with the sperm. Are there any vaginal lubricants that do not interfere?

Answer:

Petroleum jelly (such as Vaseline) is injurious to sperm. If lubrication is really necessary, the easiest is saliva. Also, certain surgical jellies which are water soluble, such as KY jelly, are minimally harmful provided only a very small amount is used.

Dear Dr. Kaufman:

Is it true that infertile couples who adopt a baby have a better chance of conceiving?

Answer:

This is a common observation in clinical practice. However, several long-term studies have failed to support the general belief that adoption increases the probability of conception in a previously infertile couple. The paradox is probably explained by the fact that many women conceive after *applying* for adoption: they then cancel the application and thus fail to appear in adoption statistics.

Dear Dr. Kaufman:

My 28-year-old daughter has been married four years and is childless by choice. I feel that no family is complete without children, but she insists that she and her husband do not plan to have any. I, in turn, feel that they probably have problems that should be looked into because of this attitude. When I mention these things to my daughter, she only gets angry. Don't you think I'm justified in my anxiety?

Answer:

Although there is an obvious desire on your part to have grandchildren, your daughter and son-in-law have the right to live their own lives and it is important to respect their wishes. Regarding problems, I would say that couples who are coerced into having children against their will often develop serious emotional problems which in turn are usually passed on to the unwanted children. In any event, even if there were serious problems, having children is certainly no solution and, on the contrary, would only bring added pressures. You'll just have to accept the idea that some couples derive more satisfaction from a childless marriage.

Dear Dr. Kaufman:

In cases where a man has weak sperm, would pooling and freezing his sperm improve his sperm quality?

Answer:

The use of frozen, pooled sperm to circumvent weak sperm or too few sperm is generally without merit. Most experts feel that semen which is incapable of producing conception under normal circumstances is not likely to survive the freezing process.

Dear Dr. Kaufman:

I have read some of your articles describing culdoscopy and laparoscopy as "look in" procedures to observe internal reproductive organs. How long ago were such examinations invented?

Answer:

The forerunners of such procedures go back at least to the time of Bozzini (1773–1809) who examined the nasal passage, the rectum, and vagina with a tubular device containing a candle light source. The results were far from satisfactory.

Over a hundred years ago, in 1869, Pantaleoni introduced hysteroscopy (looking into the uterus) as a method for the discovery of intrauterine diseases. However, it is only in the last 50 years or so that procedures were developed to examine organs *within* the body cavities.

Dear Dr. Kaufman:

Isn't it true that many women fail to conceive because they are too tense?

Answer:

In my experience, emotional tension is not the *cause* of infertility in most cases, but rather the *result* of the frustration. Many infertility problems thought to be due to emotional causes have not withstood the close scrutiny of newer diagnostic techniques.

Dear Dr. Kaufman:

Is it true that orthodox Jewish women may not have intercourse for a week following the end of their menstrual period?

Answer:

Yes, according to traditional law. The woman must count seven clean, bloodless days and is then "purified" by an immersion in a ritual bath. Only after that will she be allowed to participate in sexual relations. In most cases, this will turn out to be just about midcycle, which happens to be the most fertile time for conception. However, if her cycle is by chance shorter, or if her period lasts a lot longer than average (or if there is any intermenstrual bleeding), then intercourse might not take place near the time of ovulation, and chances of pregnancy are reduced.

FIVE

The Facts About Birth Control

Dear Dr. Kaufman:

How do you account for the continued popularity of contraceptive pills, in view of the repeated publicity about their potential danger?

Answer:

The pill has retained its popularity for the simple reason that it was the first birth control method to come along that offered an unbeatable combination: complete effectiveness, and complete freedom for sexual spontaneity. No other method has made that offer. When one does, and can add complete absence of actual or potential risk, we will be close to an "ideal" contraceptive.

Dear Dr. Kaufman:

When I stop taking the pill, will I be superfertile? I am still in my 20s.

Answer:

No, your fertility should be just about the same as it was when you started, assuming you stop within a few years and are not significantly older. Occasionally, fertility is less for a time, when there is a delay in the resumption of ovulation.

Dear Dr. Kaufman:

How soon after starting the pill is a woman protected against conception?

Answer:

In most women, protection starts from the first day of tablet taking which is on the fifth day of the menstrual cycle, counting the first day of menstruation as the first day of the cycle. However, in some women who have periods at short intervals (such as once in three weeks) ovulation may begin quite early. For such women it would be an advisable precaution to take one cycle of pills before considering themselves fully protected.

Dear Dr. Kaufman:

If my young daughter, age 7, took several of my contraceptive pills, what harm might result?

Answer:

No real harm is expected. Sometimes nausea and vomiting may result, but it passes without any need for treatment.

Dear Dr. Kaufman:

Is the contraceptive pill fully effective, even if one's periods are irregular?

Answer:

Yes. However, your doctor will undoubtedly want to know about any menstrual irregularity before prescribing the pill, in order to evaluate whether the condition needs special attention.

Dear Dr. Kaufman:

What are some of the non-serious side effects of the pill?

Answer:

Nausea, weight gain from fluid retention, tenderness of the breasts, vaginal discharge, breakthrough spotting, scanty periods—to mention the more common side effects.

Dear Dr. Kaufman:

Why is severe liver damage considered a reason *not* to take birth control pills?

Answer:

One of the functions of the liver is to detoxify estrogen. That is, the liver clears excess hormones from the blood, and if it cannot do this, such hormones can "pile up," so to speak. After liver disease, the pill (estrogen) should not be given until laboratory liver function tests have all returned to normal.

Dear Dr. Kaufman:

Can the pill be used to postpone menstruation if a woman is going on her honeymoon, or is about to have exams, or for other situations where it would be inconvenient to have a period? How is this accomplished?

Answer:

It is easily accomplished by continuing the pills for more (or fewer) days than originally scheduled.

Dear Dr. Kaufman:

My periods since taking the pill are much scantier. Does this mean that blood is being kept back which should normally be coming out?

Answer:

No. What happens is that the uterine lining doesn't develop as much as in a normal cycle, and there is consequently less loss of it during menstruation. There is no damming up of blood inside.

Dear Dr. Kaufman:

I never felt any nausea when I took the pill. Am I likely to be free from morning sickness during pregnancy when I decide to have a baby?

Answer:

That can't be predicted based only on your experience with the pill. Pregnancy is quite different.

Dear Dr. Kaufman:

How certain is it that the pill is a cause of thromboembolism? Is this now considered a scientific fact?

Answer:

It is generally accepted, though not completely, since there are enough atypical features to create some doubt.

For example, it has been observed that women in certain geographic areas such as the African tropics have virtually no thromboembolic incidents, whether or not they are on oral contraceptives. This may be because they are physically more active and slimmer than women in other countries, where thromboembolism is much more common in both pill users and non-users. There also seems to be some relationship between thromboembolism and smoking. In addition, it seems that patients with type O blood have only about one-third the incidence of thromboembolic incidents as do women with type A, B, or AB blood.

There has been a recognized increase in thromboembolism over the last ten years, beginning *before* the widespread use of the pill. Moreover, men have shown a comparable rise in thromboembolism.

For all these reasons, it is difficult to be dogmatic as to the exact relationship between the pill and thromboembolism. The classic British and American studies are widely known, and they indicate a slightly increased risk in the order of 3 deaths per 100,000 women per year for pill takers. There is also some preliminary evidence suggesting that even this figure may decrease with wider use of pills with lower estrogen content.

Dear Dr. Kaufman:

How long may birth control pills be taken? Should they be stopped every few years?

Answer:

There is no set rule, because the prescription of oral contraceptives is always on an individual basis, with continual surveillance and re-evaluation every six to twelve months. If there are no medical contraindications, the prescription may be extended indefinitely, although it would seem logical to stop altogether in the mid-40s in favor of some simpler form of contraception, as fertility is on a steep decline at that time of life.

During a woman's younger years, some doctors recommend discontinuing the pill every two years or so, to note whether spontaneous periods recur, and I think this is a good idea for any woman who intends to have children eventually. In fact, when a woman decides that she wants to start her family within a few months, the doctor may advise stopping the pill somewhat sooner, just in case there is a time lag preceding the restoration of fertility.

Dear Dr. Kaufman:

Why should the contraceptive pill be used if it is known to have certain hazards, including a mortality rate?

Answer:

It boils down to a matter of risk. Doctors, for the most part, accept the FDA estimate that the pill probably causes 3 deaths per 100,000 women per year, compared with 24 lives claimed per 100,000 annually in childbirth.

But doctors and the public constantly deal in probabilities when drugs are used. The risk of penicillin and other powerful agents is higher, but the potential benefit is great enough to make the risk widely acceptable. Most people accept far greater risks quite voluntarily. A cigarette-smoking pill taker, for example, is far more likely to die from the effects of heavy smoking than from the effects of the pill.

Dear Dr. Kaufman:

I have been on the pill for four years, and have never experienced any side effects. Would it be safe to continue taking the pill for 20 years or longer?

Answer:

Nobody knows. The longest clinical studies have been about 15 years, but the amount of scientific data is likely to be incomplete because the women taking part in the study were not originally matched with similar groups of non-users, to compare their long-term experience. It may take more than another decade to have answers, and by then we will probably have entirely different pills.

Dear Dr. Kaufman:

I have been quite happy with the pill for several months. The only unpleasant effect is some nausea, but only after the first pill. After that I feel fine. Any suggestions?

Answer:

You might start with the second pill!

Dear Dr. Kaufman:

Is there any contraceptive method even more effective than the pill?

Answer:

Total abstinence.

Dear Dr. Kaufman:

Now that the minipill is on the market, why isn't it more popular? None of my friends seem to be taking it.

Answer:

The so-called minipill has the advantage of containing no estrogenic hormone, consisting of a small dose of progestin only. Its lessened popularity is due to the fact that its effectiveness is only about 97 per cent, and there is a high incidence of irregular periods and breakthrough spotting with its use.

Dear Dr. Kaufman:

Could you explain what the contraceptive "time capsule" is?

Answer:

The "time capsule" is a silicone capsule containing progesterone, which is implanted under the skin. It releases small doses of this hormone for months. So far, experiments with rabbits and rats have been successful, and there is some work now being done with monkeys and baboons. The duration of contraceptive effect in such animals is equivalent to years in the human. Apparently, fertility is restored upon the surgical removal of the capsule.

Dear Dr. Kaufman:

What advantages does an IUD have?

Answer:

The greatest advantage may be that it is effortless. Intercourse can be spontaneous, and contraception does not depend on any action by the husband or wife. Also, it is reversible, and can easily be removed. If removal is not desired, it can remain in until normal menopause takes place.

Dear Dr. Kaufman:

If I can't feel the thread of my IUD, is there any way to tell if it has fallen out?

Answer:

When IUD threads are not felt, it most often means that the woman has not been feeling deeply enough. However, if the threads are really not detectable, the IUD may have fallen out or the threads may have been drawn up into the uterus with the IUD still in place. An examination is in order, and if the doctor confirms its absence, he will probably arrange for an x-ray or sonogram to determine whether it is in the uterus.

Dear Dr. Kaufman:

What is the historical medical background of the intrauterine device?

Answer:

About 2,000 years ago Hippocrates described a technique of inserting foreign objects for contraception into the uterus through a hollow lead tube.

In the early years of this century, a German gynecologist named Grafenberg devised a ring of coiled silver wire for intrauterine use to prevent conception. Many of his patients were unable to tolerate this device; many infections developed, and the method fell into disrepute.

However, large-scale use of various modified rings, from 1930 to 1957 in Israel and Japan, were reported to be highly successful, and this led to the development of other IUDs made of inert plastic.

Dear Dr. Kaufman:

Is it true that the longer a woman has an IUD, the less chance of pregnancy?

Answer:

Yes. The pregnancy rate does decline with time, in the case of IUD users. It is about 3 per cent the first year, about 2 per cent the second year, and about 1 per cent thereafter.

Dear Dr. Kaufman:

Under what circumstances would a physican choose not to insert an intrauterine device?

Answer:

A doctor would undoubtedly not insert an IUD if there is a known or suspected pregnancy, an inflammation in the pelvic region, a history of very painful or profuse periods, known or suspected cervical or uterine malignancy, some anatomic distortions of the uterus, and when the patient wants virtually 100 per cent contraceptive effectiveness.

Dear Dr. Kaufman:

Is an intrauterine device suitable for a young woman who has never had a child?

Answer:

With the advent of smaller and more delicate devices of different contours, such women can often be successfully accommodated with an intrauterine device. In addition, the FDA has recently released one of the copper-containing devices, thus expanding the choices that the gynecologist will have.

Dear Dr. Kaufman:

I am 32 years old and have had one child four years ago. My doctor inserted an intrauterine device a few months ago, which promptly fell out. He then suggested trying another IUD, a different kind, but I am hesitant. What are the chances of it falling out again?

Answer:

Fairly often, an IUD that has been "rejected" on one occasion may be retained on another, even the same type. It is difficult to explain why, but it's worth another try if you basically like this form of contraception.

Incidentally, if you are concerned with the possibility of the IUD falling out again, why not use a "back-up" method such as foam contraceptive *every* time you have intercourse, for the first month or so. This will give you added assurance as well as added protection. (Such foam is often advised during the most fertile days of each cycle to enhance the effectiveness rate of an IUD, and remains an option for future months.)

Dear Dr. Kaufman:

Is there a mortality rate associated with the use of intrauterine devices?

Answer:

A few years ago the American College of Obstetricians and Gynecologists surveyed its members with respect to illnesses and deaths associated with the use of IUDs. They reported four deaths traceable to the IUD itself, caused by septic infection occurring in the first week after insertion. In addition, several deaths from second trimester septic miscarriage have recently been reported in patients in whom a "shield" device had been retained.

Dear Dr. Kaufman:

If I should become pregnant while wearing an intrauterine device, can this cause a deformity in the baby? I have a "loop."

Answer:

In all such pregnancies (many have occurred) the fear of deformity in the baby has proved groundless. The reason is that the IUD lies outside the amniotic sac—that is, outside the area of the developing embryo or fetus.

Dear Dr. Kaufman:

What are the advantages and disadvantages of an IUD?

Answer:

Once an IUD has been inserted, little or no thought has to be given to contraception by either the woman or her partner. The IUD may be left in place for years. After the initial cost, there is no additional contraceptive expense (except the optional use of an additional simple method like foam during the most fertile days). Unlike the pill, IUDs exert no systemic effects on the body.

The disadvantages are that women using this method usually have a heavier flow during the first few periods after insertion. Some may complain of cramps or backache, and some may have bleeding between periods. A woman with an IUD should examine herself periodically to insure that the IUD is in place by feeling for the string. Occasionally an IUD is expelled by the uterus. Finally, this form of protection is about 97 per cent effective, unless an additional method is used during the most fertile days.

Dear Dr. Kaufman:

Why is an intrauterine device usually inserted during the menstrual period?

Answer:

There are several reasons. During a period there is more room, anatomically speaking, since the cervix dilates slightly. Secondly, it insures against inserting an IUD into a uterus which is unsuspectedly pregnant. Finally, the slight amount of bleeding that may take place during the insertion goes unnoticed at this time of the month.

Dear Dr. Kaufman:

Why do some women have trouble with an IUD, while others do not? I personally have had no difficulty but know of many women who have. Are such problems common?

Answer:

In some instances, difficulties with an IUD are almost predictable. For example, a woman with heavy periods is likely to have this feature aggravated by an IUD, and one with chronic pelvic disease is also likely to suffer recurrence of pain and other symptoms. That is why a careful medical history and physical examination are essential before a doctor considers using this form of contraception. Other factors that have some bearing upon a woman's tolerance for an IUD are her age (older women are more tolerant of it), whether she has borne children (those who have are also more tolerant), and the type and size of IUD chosen.

Dear Dr. Kaufman:

I've heard that if you should become pregnant with an IUD in the uterus, the chances of a miscarriage are higher whether the device is left in or not. Are the chances about equal?

Answer:

Some studies have indicated that the incidence of subsequent miscarriage was higher in the group in which the IUD was left in place. Specifically, about 48 per cent aborted when the device was left in, as compared with about 30 per cent when it was removed.

Dear Dr. Kaufman:

How frequently do uterine perforations occur with an IUD?

Answer:

Statistics indicate that this is quite rare, in the order of only one case in about two thousand. Perforations are most likely caused by insertion in the wrong direction, and usually occur at the time of insertion. Occasionally they can "migrate" through at some later date.

Dear Dr. Kaufman:

Is the intrauterine device ever used for any purpose other than for contraception?

Answer:

Yes. I have used it on several occasions in cases of *infertility,* where the problem was adhesions within the uterine cavity. In these cases the adhesions are broken up under anesthesia and an intrauterine device is inserted for a few months, which helps prevent the reforming of adhesions. The condition is known medically as uterine synechiae.

Dear Dr. Kaufman:

Is it possible for an intrauterine device to fall out without the woman's being aware of it?

Answer:

It's possible. Frequently there are a few signs, but of such minimal nature that the woman is unaware of what's happening.

I recently had an amusing phone call from a patient who said that she had just received a routine card from my office indicating that she was due for her annual visit. No sooner had she read it when she felt a slight cramp, and found that her IUD had fallen out. She wanted to know whether they self-destruct in one year!

Dear Dr. Kaufman:

I have an intrauterine device and also use foam during my most fertile days at the midcycle for added protection. Is the method I'm using as effective as the diaphragm with cream or jelly?

Answer:

To answer your question, certain assumptions have to be made: first, that the diaphragm was correctly fitted and that you were taught how to use it properly; and second, that the diaphragm is used every time you have intercourse. Under those conditions, the diaphragm method has a slight edge, in my opinion, since the intrauterine device, by itself, carries a pregnancy risk of perhaps 2-3 per cent. The addition of foam would certainly tend to lower that risk, however. It would be pretty close.

Dear Dr. Kaufman:

How effective is the diaphragm for contraception?

Answer:

In any individual case, the diaphragm/jelly technique is extraordinarily effective, giving virtually *complete* protection against pregnancy to those women *who are carefully and properly taught the method and use it consistently.* If one considers mass statistics—that is, countless doctors teaching countless patients the diaphragm/jelly technique—then there will be a "failure rate" of at least 5-10 per cent, or more. Even so, it is not possible to separate failures due to the method itself from failures due to incomplete or poorly understood instructions, irregular use of the method, or non-use.

Few people realize that the actual function of the diaphragm is to keep the contraceptive jelly in proper place, which is covering the cervix. Many doctors advise placing the contraceptive jelly or cream on both sides of the diaphragm (as well as around the rim) as a double line of defense.

Dear Dr. Kaufman:

What are the advantages and disadvantages of the diaphragm method of contraception?

Answer:

The advantages are that women who use the diaphragm need only concern themselves about being protected at those times when they expect to have intercourse. The diaphragm need not be inserted just before intercourse; it can be several hours before, and protection will still be there. The woman and her partner do not feel the diaphragm at all when it is properly in place. The woman need not bother to douche or remove the diaphragm right after intercourse (in fact, it should be left in place for at least six hours, and douching is unnecessary). If properly cared for, the same diaphragm may be used for at least two years, and the cost is relatively low.

The disadvantages are that the woman must first be measured by a doctor for the proper size. The diaphragm and contraceptive jelly or cream must be used whenever intercourse takes place. And some women have an aversion to inserting the diaphragm into the vagina; they obviously would not be happy with this method.

Dear Dr. Kaufman:

I am confused about one particular aspect of the diaphragm method of birth control. On the one hand, I have read that it is a very effective method if used consistently. On the other hand, I have also read that some studies indicate that during sexual activity, the "vaginal barrel" widens and elongates, causing the diaphragm to move around and making it an uncertain mechanical barrier. Thus it appears that it is not such a safe method after all. Am I right in drawing this conclusion?

Answer:

You are only right in the conclusion that the diaphragm can shift position (slightly), but wrong in the conclusion that it is not every effective. The confusion arises because many people think of the diaphragm as protecting by mechanical action. That is not its purpose.

The purpose of a diaphragm is to keep the contraceptive jelly in proper place—that is, covering the cervix. A well fitted diaphragm may shift slightly but does not move altogether off the cervix, hence the jelly continues to cover the cervix. Remember that the jelly or cream is the active spermicidal ingredient, and the diaphragm was never meant to be "air tight." One of the reasons that the doctor should choose the *largest* size that fits comfortably is to allow for spontaneous shifting within the vagina, yet maintaining cervical coverage.

Dear Dr. Kaufman:

I have used a diaphragm-with-inserter method of contraception for years. My sister recently was fitted with a diaphragm, and her doctor told her she could not use an inserter with it. Could you explain why?

Answer:

Some diaphragms, specifically the "arc" type, are so made that they cannot stretch on to an inserter, and must therefore be put in by hand. This does not make them inferior in any way, just different.

Dear Dr. Kaufman:

Suppose I forget to take my diaphragm out for several days. Could it cause infection?

Answer:

A diaphragm which is forgotten for several days is not apt to cause infection, but would almost certainly produce an irritating and offensive discharge.

Dear Dr. Kaufman:

Could constant use of the contraceptive diaphragm cause cancer in women?

Answer:

There has never been any evidence for such a relationship.

Dear Dr. Kaufman:

When was the vaginal contraceptive diaphragm first used?

Answer:

The history is a little vague, but in the 18th century Casanova mentions a partially squeezed half lemon used for this purpose. In 1838 a German gynecologist, F.A. Wilde, devised the original cervical rubber cap, to be worn from the end of one menstrual period to the beginning of the next. The modification that we recognize today as the common "diaphragm" was devised by another gynecologist, Dr. William Mensinga, in the early 1880's. It was first popularized in Holland, then brought into England and other European countries.

In 1915, Margaret Sanger, who made birth control her life's work, spent time in Holland. Upon her return to this country, she brought with her the vaginal diaphragm. When she established the first birth control clinic here in 1923, the diaphragm was the chief method of contraception offered.

Dear Dr. Kaufman:

What are the most common errors that women make in the use of the diaphragm, resulting in unplanned pregnancies?

Answer:

The most common error I have encountered is non-use of the method. With respect to the diaphragm itself, errors are failure to feel the cervix to make sure it is covered; failure to put adequate spermicide on both sides and around the rim; not putting it in at the proper time or removing it too early; and failure to have periodic check-ups to insure that the size and technique of insertion are both correct.

Dear Dr. Kaufman:

How often should I get a new diaphragm? How long does one normally last?

Answer:

Although a diaphragm may "last" for several years, it is generally advisable to get a new one about every two years. In addition, it is wise to check at regular intervals to be sure your diaphragm is in good condition.

Dear Dr. Kaufman:

I expect to get a diaphragm soon, as I intend to be married in a few months. Will I need a new size shortly after I am married?

Answer:

If a girl has not had previous sexual relations, her first diaphragm will in all probability have to be changed for a larger one within two or three months. Then her size will probably stay the same until she has had a child, at which time a change to a still larger size might be anticipated.

Dear Dr. Kaufman:

I would like a contraceptive method that is free of hazards (such as the diaphragm) but do not want to be bothered with having to put something in or take something out, before and after sex. Is there such a method?

Answer:

Yes, there is. It is called a cervical cap, and has been in use for many years, though not widely. The cervical cap is a rather sophisticated method; it consists of a plastic or aluminum cup that looks like a large thimble. The doctor fits it over the cervix, where it can remain for the entire month, to be removed during the menstrual period and then put on the cervix again when the period is over. It is essential that the size be just right, as it works on a suction principle. Once "fitted," some women can be taught to place it on their own cervix themselves, in which case it becomes a practical method of contraception. I want to emphasize again that the fit must be very good, and that the patient be instructed to make sure that the cap is firmly on the cervix, since it has the potential at least of becoming dislodged by vigorous coitus.

Dear Dr. Kaufman:

I have much difficulty with a diaphragm. Would it really be a significant risk to use spermicidal jelly alone?

Answer:

It is taking a risk to rely on spermicidal jellies, creams, or foams alone, as it is almost impossible to be sure they are covering the opening to the womb at the moment of ejaculation. If, however, you decide to take that risk, the best spermicides to use (alone) are the aerosol foams, which appear to have greater adherence.

Dear Dr. Kaufman:

I have heard that vaginal contraceptive foams or jellies by themselves are not as reliable as mechanical methods such as the condom or diaphragm. Is this true? If so, why?

Answer:

It is true. The reason chemical methods of contraception are not completely reliable is that there is no assurance that the product will be covering the opening of the womb at the crucial moment of ejaculation. Mechanical methods, on the other hand, do assure such coverage. Chemical methods, such as foams, creams, or jellies (used alone) are certainly preferable to no method at all and, with some luck, afford a moderately high degree of protection against conception in many cases.

Dear Dr. Kaufman:

I am 46 and can only use the rhythm method of birth control. However, my periods are now irregular, and I have even skipped on occasion. I always worry about being pregnant at such times. Is there any way I can regulate my cycle to make rhythm more effective?

Answer:

Whatever the age of a woman, if the menstrual cycle is irregular, rhythm becomes quite unreliable. Women in their middle and late forties characteristically start skipping periods due to fluctuating hormonal levels at this time of life. The only way you could regulate your cycle would be with hormonal medication such as contraceptive pills, which I assume are unacceptable to you. As a consolation, however, the chances of conceiving at your age are very slim and decrease even more sharply with each passing year.

Dear Dr. Kaufman:

What are the advantages and disadvantages of the rhythm method of contraception?

Answer:

The advantages are that there is no expense and no special equipment or drugs. The disadvantages are that its success depends on accurate prediction of the time when a woman releases an egg. No absolutely certain system for doing this has yet been devised. The method also restricts the number of days in which a woman can safely have intercourse. Women who menstruate irregularly cannot rely on this method at all.

Dear Dr. Kaufman:

I will be married in a few months and we plan to use the rhythm method. My doctor wants me to keep basal temperature graphs for several months which, he says, are necessary to plot my safe period. However, I am as regular as clockwork, every 28 days, and fail to see the need for keeping a daily temperature record. Couldn't the same information be given by knowing my menstrual interval, since the safe period is just an estimate anyway?

Answer:

Theoretically, yes, but from the practical point of view it would be helpful to see what your ovulatory pattern actually is, rather than to guess. I am reminded of one patient who also balked at taking temperatures. Ironically, when she finally did, it turned out that she didn't ovulate at all! She would have been using "rhythm" unnecessarily.

Dear Dr. Kaufman:

Can you please explain how the "rhythm" method derived its name?

Answer:

The method gets its name from the fact that there are alternating fertile and infertile phases in a woman's menstrual cycle. In practice, it consists of avoiding coitus at any time that might be considered fertile (near ovulation). Since pinpointing ovulation is very difficult, there must be a sufficient allowance for error, and therefore quite a few days, particularly *before* expected ovulation, are deemed unsafe. The unsafe segment continues until at least 2-3 days after the anticipated ovulation.

Dear Dr. Kaufman:

What, in your opinion, would be an ideal contraceptive?

Answer:

The ideal contraceptive is still being searched for and, when found, will be: completely effective, readily reversible, psychologically (and theologically) acceptable to all, and of course completely free of any side effects. The reason such a contraceptive does not yet exist is because complete perfection does not yet exist.

Dear Dr. Kaufman:

What is the most common form of birth control in the world?

Answer:

Withdrawal prior to ejaculation (coitus interruptus). It is the oldest and most common method used.

Dear Dr. Kaufman:

Is it true that the withdrawal technique of contraception may fail because of sperm present in the pre-ejaculatory fluid?

Answer:

This may be one reason for failure. Another reason, which most individuals do not think of, is the fact that reinsertion of the penis after ejaculation (even an hour or more later) is even more apt to contain sperm than the pre-ejaculatory fluid.

Dear Dr. Kaufman:

I read somewhere that there are several male methods of contraception, but I thought the condom was the only one. What would the others be?

Answer:

One is withdrawal, or coitus interruptus. Another is coitus reservatus, in which the man deliberately avoids reaching a climax altogether.

Dear Dr. Kaufman:

I would be interested in knowing when the condom first came into use. How effective a contraceptive is it?

Answer:

The historical background of the condom is most interesting. It was originally worn by *women* rather than men; that is, in the form of loose pouches made from animal membrane lining the vagina. The *male* condom was devised in the sixteenth century by the Italian anatomist Fallopius (the Fallopian tubes are named after him); it was a linen sheath for the penis, which he recommended for use as protection against venereal disease. Such condoms were used mainly in brothels and did not come into general use until some 300 years later, with the vulcanization of rubber.

Today, rubber condoms are used by millions throughout the world. American manufactured condoms are made either of animal membrane or latex rubber. The animal membrane that is used comes from the intestine of a sheep, imported mainly from New Zealand and Australia. They are called skin condoms and provide a higher degree of sensitivity, but are considerably more expensive. The latex rubber kind, of which most condoms are made, is similar to the rubber used in the manufacture of balloons and rubber gloves.

Condoms are available dry or lubricated. Most users prefer lubricated brands, which facilitate entry and decrease chances of breakage. Quality control in the United States is supervised by the FDA.

Regarding size—there are few significant differences in size among U.S. brands, except that skin condoms are larger because they will not stretch. Japanese condoms have been available in different *colors* for many years.

As a contraceptive, the condom used in combination with vaginal spermicide has an extremely high degree of effectiveness. In addition, it aids in the prevention of venereal disease, as well as the transmission of trichomonas, a common cause of vaginal irritation in women.

There are several objections to condoms. First, the condom must be applied prior to intercourse. This is generally annoying and disruptive to both partners. Condoms may also blunt the transmission of sensation for both partners. In addition, there is the possibility of the condom's slipping off or breaking, which can lead to unwanted pregnancy.

Dear Dr. Kaufman:

I have heard that many condoms are duds. Is there any way of testing whether they are leakproof?

Answer:

You can blow up a rubber condom in the same way as a balloon and hold it under water, which will detect even the slightest hole. Unfortunately, this test cannot guarantee infallibility since most condoms "fail" by breakage through frictional force rather than because of barely perceptible holes.

Dear Dr. Kaufman:

I wonder if there is anything new regarding contraceptive pills for men?

Answer:

The male has been relatively neglected in the field of contraceptive research, part of the difficulty being the obtaining of "volunteers." Most of the investigation regarding birth control pills for men has been conducted with prison inmates. Acutally several drugs have been found to markedly diminish sperm production to the point of clinical sterility. However, there are some serious drawbacks. Aside from taking a long time to work—sometimes weeks—the drugs being tested were associated with such unacceptable side effects as diminished sex drive and complete intolerance to alcohol in any form.

There is further research ongoing. More recently, a promising contraceptive pill is being investigated (in rats) wherein sperm, though produced, are incapable of fertilization. It is not yet known how this compound works, but one theory is that it interferes with sperm maturation in some portion of the testicle.

In point of fact, it has been the male who traditionally assumed responsibility for birth control—by withdrawal or the use of the condom. Now there is a swing back to the male after many years of women's carrying the responsibility with diaphragms, jellies, IUDs and, of course, pills.

Dear Dr. Kaufman:

What's happened to the ominous predictions regarding the population explosion? I've heard very little about it lately.

Answer:

Well, let's consider. When America was discovered only 500 years ago there were just 250 million people on the entire planet! Today, only 500 years later, the world's population is pushing 4 billion and is going to *double* by the year 2,000. Barring any major changes, 100 years from now there will be about 24 billion people on earth!

Dear Dr. Kaufman:

I have seen the slogan, in association with Planned Parenthood, "children by choice, not chance." Isn't this a kind of over-simplification of a very complex problem dealing with human reproduction?

Answer:

Any slogan is, in a sense, an over-simplification, but I am glad you asked the question. What the slogan means is that every child should be a wanted child—that pregnancy should be a planned and joyful event, never "compulsory." It means that birth control information and services should be available to all sexually active persons regardless of economic or marital status, sex, or age. In short, it means that parenthood is a personal choice.

SIX

Permanent Contraception: Sterilization

Dear Dr. Kaufman:

I understand that there are several different procedures by which a woman can be sterilized. Could you mention what they are?

Answer:

The approaches which involve *minor* surgery are as follows: (1) *Laparoscopy:* the visualization of tubes through a special instrument (laparoscope) inserted through the abdomen. A second instrument, inserted either through the laparoscope or through a separate incision, is used to close the tubes by electric current or by applying special clips. (2) *Culdoscopy:* the visualization of the tubes through a special instrument (culdoscope) which is inserted by a puncture through the back of the vagina. The tubes are then drawn out through the original puncture and closed. (3) *Colpotomy:* cutting through the back of the vagina without the use of visualizing instruments. The incision is wide enough to permit the surgeon to pull each tube through it. He then surgically cuts and ties them. (4) *Hysteroscopy:* a relatively new technique in which a visualizing instrument is inserted directly into the uterine cavity through the cervix without any incision. The instrument moves to the area of the tubes, closing them by one of several possible techniques.

The approaches which involve *major* surgery are: (1) *Laparotomy:* cutting through the abdominal wall to reach the tubes, which can then be cut or closed by various means. (2) *Hysterectomy:* the removal of the uterus. In such instances, the sterilization is secondary to the removal of the uterus for a separate medical condition.

Dear Dr. Kaufman:

To what do you attribute the rising popularity of sterilization procedures in recent years?

Answer:

There is a trend toward smaller families, for many reasons. Among these are a couple's desire for material goods and a higher standard of living, working mothers, women's liberation and the zero population growth philosophy, and general doubts as to the blessings of parenthood.

There are also a substantial number of women in their middle twenties who have completed their families and see perhaps 20 more years of fertility ahead during which they will want sexual relations but no more babies. Aware of the side effects and disadvantages of various contraceptives, they prefer a single procedure like sterilization.

Dear Dr. Kaufman:

My husband and I are interested in a permanent method of birth control. He would like to know whether vasectomy is effective and whether it interferes with intercourse or its enjoyment.

Answer:

Vasectomy is a relatively simple operative procedure in which the two spermatic ducts which lie within the scrotum are cut and tied. "Permanent" is the right word for it, since reversibility (though sometimes successful) cannot be relied upon with present methods. Thus, vasectomy is best for those couples who are quite certain they will never wish to have another child.

There is no physical interference with intercourse. Psychological difficulties are minimal provided all the facts are well understood in advance. A urologist should be consulted for more details.

Dear Dr. Kaufman:

What are sperm banks?

Answer:

Most people are aware that *blood* banks can preserve blood for many weeks by storing it in a refrigerator. Rare types of blood are kept for years by freezing the blood and storing it in liquid nitrogen at a very low temperature (-321°F).

Sperm cells, too, have been frozen and stored at low temperatures for nearly a quarter of a century. The most common use of frozen semen is in the cattle industry. Each year calves are born from millions of cows that have been inseminated with previously frozen sperm cells. This procedure has resulted in upgrading the beef and dairy herds throughout the world.

For the past two decades pioneering physicians have

been carrying on careful medical research on the insemination of frozen semen in *humans.* These early investigations have stimulated improvements in equipment and different techniques for freezing sperm, and there is ongoing research along these lines in various parts of the country.

Dear Dr. Kaufman:

Can men contemplating vasectomy be assured that banking their sperm by freezing will guarantee future fatherhood if they so desire?

Answer:

No. It would be misleading to tell such men that storing their sperm is a guarantee that they will be able to father children many years after sterilization. No period of frozen storage (and no fresh specimen, for that matter) can guarantee fertility. Men who wish "fatherhood insurance" after a vasectomy should realize that not enough information is available to promise success. In other words, a man desiring a vasectomy should consider the procedure permanent.

Dear Dr. Kaufman:

If a woman is sterilized by having her tubes tied, will menstrual periods still continue?

Answer:

Yes. The womb and ovaries are unchanged by the operation. The ovaries continue to release an egg each month. Tying the tubes merely prevents the egg from moving into the womb.

Dear Dr. Kaufman:

I have heard that sterilization procedures in women can be done by cauterization without going into the abdominal cavity. How is this possible?

Answer:

You are probably referring to a relatively new experimental method—cauterization (burning) of the inner opening to the tubes where they join the uterus. This can be done by inserting a special instrument through the cervix into the uterus, and cauterizing the utero-tubal juncture. It is done under local anesthesia, with prior dilatation of the cervix to permit the introduction of the special instrument, called a hysteroscope.

X-rays of the uterus and tubes are taken at several-month intervals to determine whether tubal closure has occurred. During this waiting time the patient continues with whatever contraceptive method she has been using.

The procedure has not yet been used widely enough to permit large statistical studies for evaluation, particularly long-term follow up.

Dear Dr. Kaufman:

Can tying the tubes affect a woman's sexual drive or response?

Answer:

From the anatomical and physiological standpoint, no, since sexual satisfaction is a cerebral rather than genital function. From an emotional point of view, however, it would depend on how much counseling and screening there was prior to sterilization.

Not surprisingly, when patients are well screened, follow-up reports have been quite favorable. A closer look at patients who react poorly postoperatively often reveals a subconsicous need either to have another baby, or at least feel that they *could* have another baby.

The attitude of the husband is also important. Some men are very supportive, but others insist the decision be made entirely by the wife, often leaving her bewildered. Some husbands may even become hostile after the procedure, with a feeling that their wives are less feminine since they cannot bear children. They may also feel that they themselves are less masculine since they cannot "prove" their masculinity by impregnating their wives. Careful screening as well as counseling would presumably alert the physician or counselor to such attitudes and feelings and mitigate against performing the procedure, after proper explanations.

Dear Dr. Kaufman:

I understand that the testicles not only produce sperm, but also manufacture the male hormone. If my husband should have a vasectomy, which we are considering, would this interfere with hormonal production?

Answer:

No. The cells which produce the male hormone testosterone continue to be as active as before the operation.

Dear Dr. Kaufman:

I am 64 and my husband is 68. He has had difficulty obtaining an erection in the past two years, and wondered if the sterilization operation (vasectomy) will help him in this respect.

Answer:

I regret to say that it will not.

SEVEN

Abortion

Dear Dr. Kaufman:

Has it ever been calculated what the risk is of pregnancy occurring with a single unprotected exposure?

Answer:

For a single *random* exposure, the risk is about 3 per cent. However, if the single exposure is during the five or so most fertile days of the cycle, the risk jumps to between 15–20 per cent.

Dear Dr. Kaufman:

How safe are abortions after the 12th week as compared with those performed during the first three months?

Answer:

A large scale national survey indicated that, even in the best of hands, the incidence of major medical complications from abortions performed in advanced pregnancies ("saline abortions") is at least four times as great as in early pregnancy. This is but one of several reasons why women who plan to terminate pregnancy should seek help during the first three months. Incidentally, this survey also indicated that the incidence of *major* medical complications during the first three months was only 0.5 per cent.

Dear Dr. Kaufman:

How does the mortality rate from legal abortion in New York City compare to the low mortality rate from the same procedure in various European countries where abortion has been legal for many years?

Answer:

In some Eastern European countries, almost all abortions are performed only in the first trimester, and very low mortality ratios have been reported for a number of years. For example, in Hungary the ratio was 2.2 deaths per 100,000 abortions. In Czechoslovakia the ratio was 2.8 deaths per 100,000 procedures. Although these very low rates have sometimes been questioned by Western observers, they have now been confirmed by the New York experience.

The overall mortality with legal abortion in New York City between 1970 and 1972 was 5.0 deaths per 100,000 legal abortions, but this included both first *and* second trimester cases. The mortality rate was nine times higher in the second trimester as compared with the first trimester.

Dear Dr. Kaufman:

How is an abortion performed during the first twelve weeks?

Answer:

Under either local or general anesthesia, the upper lip of the cervix is grasped, the cervix is gradually dilated (usually after sounding the depth of the uterus), and then the uterine contents are evacuated by suction, followed by curettage (scraping) to insure complete removal of all fragments.

Dear Dr. Kaufman:

What exactly is done in a saline abortion?

Answer:

A saline abortion, or so-called "salting out" procedure is done from about the 16th week of pregnancy to the 20th week. Most hospitals will not accept a patient after the 20th week, as the likelihood of a live birth is greater after that time.

A saline abortion is performed by inserting a needle through the abdominal wall after injecting a local anesthetic. The doctor draws out a certain amount of amniotic fluid surrounding the fetus and replaces it with salt solution. This results in uterine contractions and, finally, the expulsion of a non-living fetus—that is, a miscarriage.

The patient may have to be hospitalized up to three days because the time lag between the salt injection and the expulsion of the fetus varies from six to seventy-two hours.

Dear Dr. Kaufman:

I've read somewhere that seaweed has been used for abortion in certain countries. Is this true?

Answer:

Yes, the substance used is known as a "laminaria tent," and it is an efficient means for cervical dilatation, particularly before suction curettage in young women.

Laminaria is a species of seaweed. When dry, the stem is capable of expanding to three to five times its original diameter. It is actually an old technique, and modern autoclaving methods have rendered some of the old objections invalid. The slow dilatation and cervical softening accomplished by the tent spares the patient much trauma and blood loss, according to its advocates.

The procedure consists of inserting a sterile laminaria tent into the cervix. The patient then returns in 24 hours for a suction abortion. Very often, no further dilatation of the cervix is required. The procedure has been quite popular in Great Britain, Germany, Japan, and several other countries.

Dear Dr. Kaufman:

What is the most common delayed complication of abortion?

Answer:

Possibly prematurity in subsequent births. The chances of such subsequent premature births increases with each induced abortion. Whether this tendency is related to cervical weakening or to the increased age and number of pregnancies of the patient (or still other factors) is not definitely known.

Dear Dr. Kaufman:

What exactly is menstrual regulation? Is it the same as menstrual extraction?

Answer:

The procedure goes by various names: menstrual regulation, menstrual extraction, menstrual induction, mini-suction, mini-abortion, and so on. The reason for the term "menstrual regulation" is that before the Supreme Court overthrew restrictive state abortion laws, the procedure was intended to be used before a pregnancy test was positive, and when the only "sign" of pregnancy was a missed period; hence the term "regulation."

It is important to be aware of the possibility of a continued pregnancy if it fails, and obviously a certain number of non-pregnanct women will have undergone the procedure needlessly. Local anesthesia is required in about one fourth of patients undergoing this procedure.

By whatever name, the operation is basically an abortion, except that it is done at such an early stage that the woman is not sure she is pregnant.

Dear Dr. Kaufman:

Some feminist groups have been extracting each others' menses each month. I'd like to know how this is done, and your opinion of the whole procedure.

Answer:

Three benefits are claimed by feminist groups advocating this procedure: no need for contraceptives, the elimination of several days of menstrual bleeding, and the termination of a very early pregnancy if one has conceived. In the latter instance, the procedure is clearly an early abortion.

One might ask advocates of this procedure how they would regard it if a group of *men* advised a procedure they had only been experimenting with a short time (with no additional information about side effects or hazards) and recommended that women experiment with each other. There would no doubt be accusations of irresponsibility.

The fact of the matter is that we do not know what long-term effects of such a procedure would be. If carried out monthly there is also at least the potential danger of perforation, infection, and subsequent sterility.

Dear Dr. Kaufman:

What is the overall risk of complications from first trimester abortions in the United States?

Answer:

According to a study conducted by Dr. Christopher Tietze, Associate Director of the Biomedical Division of the Population Council, the incidence of minor medical complications in the first trimester was one in twenty. The risk of major complications associated with legal first-trimester abortions was one in two hundred. These major complications included all patients receiving unintended major surgery during this time (such as repair of a perforated uterus, or a hysterectomy or hysterotomy), or patients given a blood transfusion, or patients with three or more days of fever or other categories connected with long illness or functional impairment.

Dear Dr. Kaufman:

Is it true that there is greater risk of miscarriage in later pregnancies if one has had an induced abortion?

Answer:

The termination of a pregnancy by dilatation of the cervix may indeed increase the risk of a spontaneous miscarriage during the second trimester of a subsequent pregnancy, according to some studies. This is apparently due to some weakening of the cervix, which causes a premature dilatation. There does not seem to be any increased incidence of first trimester spontaneous miscarriages following an induced abortion.

Dear Dr. Kaufman:

I assume that perforation of the uterus is one of the most dreaded complications of an abortion. How often does this occur?

Answer:

In one of the largest free-standing clinics in New York there was an analysis of a total of 30,000 abortions performed between February 1, 1971 and March 31, 1972. Of the 30,000 abortions, there were 24 documented uterine perforations, an incidence of less than one (0.8) per 1,000. This compares favorably with the statistics reported from other large facilities.

Dear Dr. Kaufman:

I wonder if you could settle an argument. I understand that the use of suction for removing uterine contents is not new but can be traced to Japanese sources some years ago. A friend says that the original work was done in Russia even before that, perhaps 15 or 20 years ago. Who is right?

Answer:

Actually, neither is right. The suction principle in obstetrics and gynecology was in use as long ago as the 17th century! The use of this principle for *diagnostic* aspiration-curettage was also described by the well known gynecologist, Emil Novak, in 1935, and he made no claims for originality.

Dear Dr. Kaufman:

Am I correct in assuming that drugs like prostaglandins, which induce abortion chemically, would eliminate all the hazards of surgical abortion?

Answer:

No. It is true that the major complications of surgical abortion are related to the surgical nature of the procedure —that is, hemorrhage, uterine perforation, or infection. However, in looking over the development of drug-induced abortion, one must keep in mind that with the exception of uterine perforation, many complications are simply inherent in the process of reproduction. Thus, hemorrhage and infection still are possible, not to mention side effects from the drug itself that is used to induce abortion. Possibly the greatest area of need for a non-surgical approach to abortion is between the 13th and 16th week of pregnancy, when the patient is too large for a standard surgical abortion and too early for a saline abortion. Similarly, beyond the 16th week prostaglandins may eventually replace the salting-out procedure altogether.

Dear Dr. Kaufman:

When I discussed having an abortion with my doctor he said he would prefer to wait about two more weeks, as I was too early in my pregnancy. Is it not true, however, that the best time to perform an abortion is as early as possible?

Answer:

No, not necessarily. In a very large and well documented study on abortion, it was found that complications, especially major ones, were higher for abortions performed at six weeks' gestation or less than at seven to ten weeks' gestation. This may sound paradoxical, but is explained by the fact that in a woman who is pregnant for the first time, the cervix is generally very rigid and tight; it is easier to injure or perforate such a cervix in an attempted abortion. Waiting a week or two longer permits the cervix to soften up and then dilatation is easier, as there is less resistance.

Dear Dr. Kaufman:

Why is it that some authorities insist on calling endometrial aspiration an abortion if the woman is only 2-3 days overdue and the pregnancy test is negative?

Answer:

It is true that in such cases the status of pregnancy has not been definitely established. More accurately, then, endometrial aspiration might be defined as an abortion if a woman happens to be pregnant, and an unnecessary procedure if she is not.

Dear Dr. Kaufman:

What exactly is the morning-after pill? How does it work? How effective is it? Are there any serious side effects?

Answer:

There is no such thing as a specific morning-after pill, since the term can apply to any form of high estrogen medication which is prescribed the "morning after" exposure to pregnancy (actually within 72 hours after such exposure). The estrogen may be in the form of an injection, pills, or both, and is continued for 4-5 days. However, most of the research has been with the synthetic estrogen, diethylstilbestrol (DES), which the FDA has recently "approved" for this purpose under "emergency" circumstances.

Since such treatment does not interfere with fertilization, it is believed that the mechanism of action is by somehow interfering with implantation.

When large doses of estrogen are used, the effectiveness is believed to be very great. However, exact statistics are difficult to come by, for several reasons. For one thing, the fertility of the patient or her partner is often unknown. Furthermore, the validity of the exposure is not always reliable; there may have been more than one exposure. Nor is the medication always taken as directed.

Side effects are usually more annoying than serious, with nausea and vomiting being the most predominant. Less frequently, there may be headache, dizziness, menstrual irregularity or breast soreness. There is also a question as to whether estrogens will have an adverse effect on the fetus if given in ineffective doses or after implantation. Since such effects are presently unknown, it is very important to explain that if there is failure, abortion is advisable.

Dear Dr. Kaufman:

Is it true that the so-called morning-after pill accomplishes its purpose by abortion?

Answer:

Medically speaking, no. A better term is interception. The so-called morning-after pill, which is high dosage estrogen, does not interfere with fertilization and will not interrupt an established implantation. Therefore it can not be defined either as a contraceptive or an abortifacient. The medication can, however, intercept a fertilized egg before it implants. Interception may be defined as the process of preventing implantation after unprotected coitus.

EIGHT

All About Sex

Dear Dr. Kaufman:

Which is anatomically more sensitive, the penis or the clitoris?

Answer:

The clitoris has more nerve endings than the penis. Embryologically we were all females until the sixth week of gestation.

Dear Dr. Kaufman:

Does a woman produce a fluid during orgasm?

Answer:

Not necessarily during orgasm, but there is a transudate (sweat) from the vaginal wall that begins to develop during sexual excitation.

Dear Dr. Kaufman:

Has anal eroticism always been considered an anti-social act? In our society there even seem to be laws against this type of sexual behavior.

Answer:

The social acceptability of anal sexual activity has not always been negative, and has varied in different cultures. In ancient Peru, anal intercourse between husband and wife was mandatory when she started to nurse after pregnancy, until the third year of the offspring's life. The punishment for vaginal coitus during this time was death. There is also ample evidence that anal intercourse was practiced by the ancient Greeks and Romans. However, during the middle ages anal intercourse was punishable by execution.

In modern times anal intercourse has been quite common. In this connection, the use of self-inserted objects sometimes comes to the attention of the medical profession in the form of foreign objects that have been "lost" in the rectum, requiring emergency removal. I recall one case described in the *Journal of the American Medical Association* where an x-ray in the emergency room of a hospital showed a table knife lodged in the intestine, which had obviously been inserted through the rectum. The *Journal* dryly described the patient's history, noting that his chief complaint was "knife-like pains in the abdomen."

Dear Dr. Kaufman:

What is the best aphrodisiac for men?

Answer:

A warm and receptive woman.

Dear Dr. Kaufman:

What is the difference between libido and potency in a man?

Answer:

Impotence can be defined as the inability to have or maintain an erection until ejaculation occurs. Libido means sexual desire. Thus, any man who completely lacks libido is, in fact, impotent, but every impotent man does not lack desire. In fact, it is distinctly unusual for a man to have permanent absence of sexual desire.

Dear Dr. Kaufman:

How prevalent is oral-genital contact?

Answer:

Kinsey reported that 54 per cent of couples questioned had experienced oral-genital contact, but there is evidence that since that report the incidence is much higher. It is hardly surprising that the two areas of the body that are erotically most sensitive should often be brought into direct contact. It is certainly a common practice among all classes of mammals.

Dear Dr. Kaufman:

I am too embarrassed to ask anyone this question, and am almost too shy to write it down. Is there any harm from swallowing sperm?

Answer:

None at all, provided the man does not have venereal disease, or viral herpes (a form of infectious blisters on the penis).

Dear Dr. Kaufman:

For some strange reason my husband has become worried that his penis is too small when erect, though I haven't noticed any difference in size. Besides, I am quite satisfied sexually, so I don't know why he is concerned. Are there any statistics about normal size that I can use to reassure him?

Answer:

The late Dr. Robert L. Dickinson, who was a pioneer in the field of sexology (ahead of Kinsey), became interested in the average size of various reproductive organs several decades ago, and his findings are included in his classic text, *Human Sex Anatomy.* The result of measurement in 1,500 white American males was as follows: average length of the erect penis was 6¼ inches; in 90 per cent the range was between 5 and 7½ inches; the diameter varied between 1¼ to 1½ inches. More important, it appears that size alone has little to do with sexual pleasure for either partner.

The vagina distends only for the size of the penis which is inserted. Also, most of the orgasmic muscular contractions occur in the outer third of the vagina. The exact length and width of an erect penis thus bears no relationship to the satisfaction of the female partner, other than a purely psychological one. Actually, erect penises vary very little in size, despite great apparent differences in the limp state.

Dear Dr. Kaufman:

I don't remember where I read it, but I seem to recall something about a man's growth of beard in relation to sexual stimulation. Would you have any idea what I am referring to?

Answer:

You are probably referring to a demonstration that a man who is in isolation and away from sexual opportunities has a tendency to diminished beard growth. Apparently the psyche influences the glandular function in this respect. Yes, it works the other way around too; with the return of sexual opportunity beard growth becomes more rapid again.

Dear Dr. Kaufman:

My husband frequently wishes to have sexual relations when I'm not in the mood. This often causes a conflict, and I wondered what we could do to prevent such conflicts?

Answer:

In a well adjusted marriage, each partner is eager to please the other, and the frequency of intercourse simply does not come up as a subject for debate or argument. No one is "counting."

Your own situation raises other questions, such as why are you not in the mood so often? Is your husband unreasonable in his demands? How do the two of you get along outside your bedroom? As you undoubtedly know, a woman is physically capable of participating in sex even if she is initially not in the mood; frequently the giving of pleasure is enough to change her own mood from passive acceptance to active desire. You may both want to talk over your "conflict" with an experienced counselor.

Dear Dr. Kaufman:

How can a marriage possibly be happy if the sexual relationship is poor?

Answer:

It can't be. Sex reflects the tone of a marriage, and a poor physical relationship is generally just a symptom of general marital distress.

Dear Dr. Kaufman:

What is the origin of the word "masturbation"?

Answer:

Most probably it comes from the Latin *manus* (hand) and *turbare* (to stir up); to stir up by hand.

Dear Dr. Kaufman:

All other factors being equal, isn't there a natural slowdown in sexual drive and response as one gets older?

Answer:

Sex is unique in that a sharp decline in sex drive is not really natural unless a person consciously or subconsciously wishes it to be so. The real reasons for the commonly observed decline in sex drive with advancing years have to do with such factors as chronic illness, fatigue, and plain loss of interest because of new areas of concern or stress in the lives of both partners.

Culturally, one notes, old people aren't supposed to be so frisky sexually. Note that an audience will always laugh at a play or movie where an elderly woman chides her amorous husband with "act your age." This is absurd, of course, as is readily seen when there is a remarriage of an older man or woman, with consequent resurgence of sexual drive that neither partner would have thought possible. In general, a woman's libido after menopause is very much influenced by her sexual patterns premenopausally. While it is true that the aging male and female show slower orgasmic reaction times, this does not necessarily interfere with sexual enjoyment.

Dear Dr. Kaufman:

My husband makes very few sexual demands on me, which suits me fine. However, I'm beginning to wonder whether I should be worried?

Answer:

The wife who says, "I have a very considerate husband; he never bothers me. . ." is revealing a great deal about her relationship. And so is the woman who just tolerates sex with an "all right, if you must" attitude. Whether or not you should be worried (presumably about extramarital affairs on your husband's part) is something only you can answer, since you know him best.

Dear Dr. Kaufman:

I've never had the courage to indulge in anal intercourse, and wondered what possible advantage it would have for a woman. What is the possibility of infection?

Answer:

For some women the anus may be an erogenous area. In some older women whose vaginas are so stretched from childbirth that there is a lack of muscle tone, anal entry might be viewed as compensatory. In addition, there is, of course, the advantage of its being a sure method of contraception.

On the other hand, anal (rectal) intercourse can be quite painful if there is spasm, and therefore careful lubrication and gentleness are essential. Even so, injury sometimes results in a fissure, or aggravates previously existing rectal conditions such as hemorrhoids.

Hygienic precautions should be observed to avoid the possibility of infection. The rectum should be empty, and the penis must be carefully washed afterward if there is to be any subsequent vaginal entry. If the female has rectal gonorrhea, it will in all probability be transmitted to the male, and vice versa. The use of a condom would eliminate most of these risks.

Dear Dr. Kaufman:

I am subject to recurrent vaginal irritation, itching, and discharge and wondered whether oral-genital contact could be causing these recurrences.

Answer:

The two most common causes of vaginal irritation, itching, and discharge are trichomonas (a harmless parasite), and monilia (a fungus, or yeast). The trichomonas organism has not been isolated from the mouth and therefore presumably is not transmitted during cunnilingus. Monilia (fungus, yeast) can colonize in the mouth and presumably could be transmitted from the mouth to the vagina during oral-genital contact. However, if monilia is cultured from the mouth, there is the question of whether it was transmitted from the vagina, rather than the other way around. Also, normal bacterial flora in the vagina usually (but not always) prevent overgrowth of monilia. In any event, it is simple enough to take cultures for monilia from the mouth of both partners to see if such transmission is at least a possibility. The eradication of symptomless monilia from the mouth involves rinses with an anti-fungicide solution for a few days.

Dear Dr. Kaufman:

It is common knowlege that bidets are used throughout many European countries but are relatively rare in the United States. Is it that they are of little value, or are we lagging behind the times in hygienic matters?

Answer:

The basin equipped with a built in spray, known as the bidet, is indeed popular in some European countries, especially in France. It is used in the morning and evening, always after defecation, and before intercourse. Its users feel that any other method of genital and anal cleansing is not adequate.

In the United States we have substituted a daily shower or bath, presumably with careful attention to the genitals and anus too. However, there is no question but that dry toilet paper after defecation is an inadequate (and irritating) cleanser, and is not as effective as moistened toilet paper or a hygienic towelette.

Dear Dr. Kaufman:

My husband and I are middle aged, and for some time now I have been troubled by vaginal discomfort whenever we try to have intercourse. This is most distressing, as we love each other very much, and I would like to fulfill our mutual desires. What could be wrong?

Answer:

You should be examined to see if there is some local irritation that can be cleared up. Often the cause is simply a thinning of the vaginal tissues, due to diminished estrogenic hormone in that area, which is a common condition in older women. If this is the case, the application of an estrogenic cream (a prescription drug) dramatically reverses the process and makes intercourse comfortable and pleasurable again.

Dear Dr. Kaufman:

In your experience, has the common use of tampons reduced the incidence of painful intercourse during the first sexual encounter?

Answer:

The widespread use of tampons for menstrual protection has indeed reduced the chances of discomfort during first intercourse. One reason is that there is a gradual stretching of the hymen. In addition, frequent use of tampons minimizes reflex muscular "protective" spasms which could create discomfort.

Dear Dr. Kaufman:

I have been told that it is not necessary or advisable to douche. However, I like to do so rather frequently, almost daily, because I feel it keeps me cleaner. I use either plain water or water to which I have added a little vinegar. My question is: even though it may not be necessary, am I doing myself any harm by frequent douching?

Answer:

Medical concern about the possible adverse effects of frequent vaginal douching are based on the premise that there is an alteration of vaginal bacteria and a consequent changing of the normal acidity. However, in one rather comprehensive study of women who douched daily with various acid and alkaline solutions, it was found that there were no changes in vaginal acidity as measured electronically. Nor were there any changes in the cell structure of the vaginal mucous membrane, as determined by Pap smears.

Of course, if a person douches with undiluted or strong substances, severe irritation may result. Also, allergic-type reactions have been noted by some users of perfumed and "flavored" douches.

In short, although it is true that normally the vagina does not require douching for cleanliness, it also seems to be true that douching with *mild* substances is generally harmless. Therefore, while I do not encourage a woman to douche "routinely," neither do I discourage those women who, for personal reasons, desire to do so.

Dear Dr. Kaufman:

My husband is 51 and seems to be despondent over the fact that he cannot achieve an erection as often as he used to. This doesn't disturb me much, but I can see how upset it makes him. I wonder what advice can be given.

Answer:

After ruling out organic illness or emotional disturbance, the first step might be to explain that there may be a natural slowdown with age, and that any man falls into a trap if he begins to keep score on successes and "failures." It should also be explained that there are a number of other ways to please his wife and satisfy himself, aside from intercourse. Thus, simply removing the *need* for complete erection would remove his preoccupation with sexual failure.

Dear Dr. Kaufman:

Why is there so much emphasis on sexual problems? I know they exist, but I wonder why they should be so prevalent in our society.

Answer:

In our society we have been emphasizing performance rather than pleasure. Feeling completely responsible for the response of one's partner often leads to performance failure due to anxiety. It may sound almost too simple, but when people stop emphasizing the genital area and concentrate on receiving maximal pleasure from *non-genital* physical contact, their genitals paradoxically often begin to work!

Dear Dr. Kaufman:

I don't know what it is, but although I am active all day with my children and other work, when it comes to sex at night I seem to be too tired. My husband is usually very understanding, but has become impatient recently. Could there be a psychological explanation for the way I feel?

Answer:

Because it can be so vague, fatigue is an effective disguise for sexual disharmony. Such disharmony is, in turn, a reflection of deeper marital discord. Sex avoidance can take many forms: "Not tonight, honey, I have a headache," or "I was at the beauty parlor and don't want to mess my hair," or that zinger, "All right, if you must!" response, with which any woman can torpedo a man's ardor and effectiveness.

More subtle (nonverbal) ways in which women may avoid sex are by poor personal hygiene and obesity. Obese women are often not aware that their overweight keeps sexual contact to a minimum.

Whatever mechanism is at work, it is the marriage relationship itself that must be examined in order to understand why there is a reluctance to participate in a closer physical relationship. Sex is, after all, not simply a meeting of the bodies but a form of communication which depends on a sustained atmosphere of mutual affection. It is when love declines that sex becomes a chore.

Dear Dr. Kaufman:

If my husband had his way, he would spend all of his spare time in the bedroom, and I don't mean watching television. He seems to have an insatiable desire for sex.

Answer:

There is a saying that sex is not just in the bedroom, it's in every room in the house. From what you say, the tremendous physical attraction that you apparently have for him is, for you, more exhausting than flattering. Without further information (age, years married, etc.), it would be difficult to advise. The adage that most divorces start in the bedroom stems from the fact that this is the most sensitive room in the house, and sex is an excellent barometer of a couple's relationship.

Dear Dr. Kaufman:

I have often heard it said that fear of impotence can cause the very failure in sex that is feared. But what is the psychological basis for this?

Answer:

Fear of impotence can cause failure in sex for the same reasons that fear can cause a person to become "white as a sheet." When the body feels threatened, blood is withdrawn from the external organs such as the skin (or the penis) and is concentrated on the internal organs, to minimize bleeding in case of "attack."

One of the best remedies for impotence is for the man to concentrate during sexual activity on pleasure *alone.*

Dear Dr. Kaufman:

My husband is able to have an erection and normal intercourse but cannot ejaculate during intercourse. However, he is able to masturbate to the point of ejaculation. How could this be explained?

Answer:

I have encountered a number of such instances in my own medical practice. Such cases of so-called ejaculatory impotence have no known physical basis. The obvious explanation is a subconscious wish not to impregnate, but it is probably much more complex than that. In the cases I have encountered it has not been possible to change the pattern, even with prolonged psychotherapy, and the couples have simply adjusted to the situation.

Dear Dr. Kaufman:

What are the causes of impotence?

Answer:

There are physiological, physical, and emotional causes. Physiological and physical causes are relatively uncommon, consisting of such illnesses as diabetes, some urological diseases, and certain neurological disorders. Other causes are transient, such as overindulgence in alcohol or drugs, fatigue, or poor health.

Most cases of impotence are emotional. *Chronic* impotence is difficult to remedy; it may be related to a background that is anti-sexual or anti-pleasure, possibly with an exploitative mother or a castrating father. The chief cause of *temporary* impotence is impotence itself! Any concentration on performance tends to result in continuing failure. It is especially common for men in their 40s or 50s to worry about actual or potential impotence. The fear of failure to perform up to their preconceived notions, standards, or fantasies only perpetuates the problem.

Other causes of impotence are misinformation, depression, any blow to self-esteem and, of course, changes in the interpersonal relationship of the couple.

Dear Dr. Kaufman:

My husband is 54 and I think he has a feeling that his age has made him an inferior sexual partner as compared to younger men. I feel sure this is not true. Is age a significant factor?

Answer:

There is a lot of brainwashing in our culture to the effect that older people are not sexually attractive or capable, which can have a devastating emotional impact on any man who believes it. The fact is, age does play a role, but not necessarily a detrimental one! Men between the ages of 50 and 70 can actually have better control of ejaculation than younger men, which is an advantage. On the other hand, it is also true that older men attain an erection more slowly and orgasm may not last as long as it did in the past. There is also a decrease in the amount of seminal fluid produced.

None of these changes brings less sexual satisfaction to the man or his partner.

Dear Dr. Kaufman:

Would you happen to know why the rhinoceros horn remains in great demand as a reputed aphrodisiac?

Answer:

One would think it is because of its phallic symbolism, but there is a more logical explanation. Those knowledgeable in the habits of African animals point out that the duration of coitus of the rhinoceros is probably much longer than that of other animals, lasting a half hour or more. Incidentally, the rhinoceros horn consists of compressed hair, not ivory or bone. When used as an aphrodisiac it is generally ground into a fine powder and mixed with water or wine, the "effective" dose being about a one-inch length of horn. Like most so-called aphrodisiacs, its "effectiveness" is all in the mind.

Dear Dr. Kaufman:

Some say that alcohol can be a sexual stimulant, and others disagree. What are the facts?

Answer:

Alcohol's reputation as an aphrodisiac comes from the fact that in moderate quantities it may reduce fears and guilt feelings that might otherwise interfere with sexual enjoyment or performance. In larger quantities, however, alcohol blocks the neural pathways that control erection, causing temporary impotence. Of course, a woman is capable of intercourse even when drunk, but her chances of satisfactory orgasm are diminished in that state.

Dear Dr. Kaufman:

Are human beings the only mammals to experience orgasm, or do other animals have it too?

Answer:

As far as male mammals are concerned, the answer is yes, since orgasm can be equated with ejaculation. However, I know of no conclusive evidence that female mammals definitely have orgasm. Observations indicate that some female mammals enjoy copulation during the receptive period of the cycle, while others appear indifferent.

Dear Dr. Kaufman:

Is it more sexually stimulating if partners don't see too much of each other in the nude except when they want to have sexual relations?

Answer:

This misconception may have stemmed from the early 1900s, when some women would brag that their husbands had never seen them in the nude. They would get undressed in a closet and have intercourse with nightclothes on.

On the contrary, nude sleeping is pleasurable in itself and literally tells the partner that there is no barrier between them. Obviously this is more enjoyable in a double bed.

I am reminded of a short story by de Maupassant called, I believe, *The Bed*, in which a family moves out of a house with their twin beds, and the villagers stand around to see who the new occupants will be. When they see movers bringing in a double bed, they break out in spontaneous applause.

Dear Dr. Kaufman:

Is it possible for a woman to have a partial orgasm? After reading a lot about this subject, I am more confused than ever.

Answer:

The word "partial" apparently refers to the degree of intensity of orgasm and implies that it is something less than oceanic, volcanic, mind-blowing, rocket-launching, or earth-shaking. Actually, the intensity of a woman's orgasm varies, depending upon her general mood, degree of preparation, and many other psychosexual factors. This is in marked contrast to male orgasm, which is seldom "partial."

Dear Dr. Kaufman:

My husband is a professional athlete. I've often wondered whether or not athletic performance is diminished by intercourse the night before. I've heard varying views.

Answer:

No less an authority on human sexuality than Dr. William Masters, himself a former athlete, once said in an interview that after intercourse athletes should be able to perform with maximum ability if they are allowed a sufficiently long recuperation period—one to five minutes!

Dear Dr. Kaufman:

I am troubled by diminishing sex drive after six years of marriage, with no apparent cause. I have consulted several psychologists who told me there is nothing specific they can do to help. Isn't there a hormone which can increase a woman's sex drive?

Answer:

Testosterone, the male sex hormone, tends to increase female sex drive by increasing clitoral sensitivity, but only in women whose sex drives have been normal in the past. However, it does not get to the true (emotional) causes. Obviously the physician consulted will want to know about the marital history in detail in order to determine whether such therapy might be worthwhile, at least on a trial basis. The problem of prolonged testosterone therapy is that it can produce unpleasant side effects such as acne or increased body hair.

Dear Dr. Kaufman:

I have read the works of Masters and Johnson, and they seem to indicate that orgasm is more intense by masturbation than by actual intercourse. Does this not seem paradoxical?

Answer:

Female orgasm is very complex, and "more intense" does not necessarily mean more satisfying. Most women will report that although "autoerotic" or "automanipulative" techniques, as they are referred to, cause intense orgasm, they are actually more satisfied when such orgasm is achieved during intercourse, even though the intensity may actually be less.

Dear Dr. Kaufman:

I am confused about vaginal versus clitoral orgasm—the fact that many authorities consider them identical. It seems to me that vaginal orgasm should be much more satisfying.

Answer:

The *physiological* response to female orgasm is apparently the same, no matter how produced. However, orgasm by clitoral stimulation alone, particularly if it is by masturbation, lacks intimate sharing and so the physiological response may lack the *psychological* involvement which accompanies orgasm before, during, and after intercourse.

Dear Dr. Kaufman:

I am a young husband, age 22, and we had our first child several months ago. Since then my wife has shown a noticeable disinterest in sex. What medical explanation could there be for this, as it is most distressing to me?

Answer:

"Disinterest" in sex can have many meanings, and it is essential to communicate with each other (or with a professional counselor) to uncover the meanings pertinent to your own situation. Among the possibilities, one frequently sees sexual disinterest as a subtle form of punishment, perhaps for the fact that the pregnancy was unplanned, or for consequent physical or financial stresses. Keep in mind, too, that abstinence is the "best" form of contraception, particularly if a young mother is unsure of being adequately protected against another pregnancy.

Dear Dr. Kaufman:

How often do you hear about pelvic congestion and discomfort from unsatisfied sexual arousal in female patients?

Answer:

Such pelvic discomfort is not uncommon, and on close questioning many patients will report that masturbation is often resorted to in order to relieve the discomfort from the congestion. However, we also see many women who cannot seem to relieve the discomfort by masturbation or coitus, and they commonly have such symptoms as chronic non-irritating (clear) vaginal discharge, pelvic heaviness, low backache, fatigue, irritability, and insomnia. These are some of the hidden symptoms of chronic sexual dissatisfaction.

Dear Dr. Kaufman:

Why is there still so much discussion about masturbation when it is generally accepted to be harmless?

Answer:

Because it wasn't always accepted as harmless. Viewed today, the history of attitudes toward masturbation are almost unbelievable. For many decades there were actual restraining devices in an attempt to prevent this "terrible practice." Between 1866 and 1932 the U.S. Government Patent Office awarded 33 patents to inventors of sexual restraints. The first patent for a masturbation "lock," dated June 14, 1870, bears this revealing preamble: "My invention is a device for so covering up the sexual organs of a person addicted to the vice of masturbation from his own touch and control that he or she must refrain from the commission of this vicious and self-degrading act."

Dear Dr. Kaufman:

I have often wondered how early in life children are capable of orgasm.

Answer:

From about the fifth month of life. The word orgasm, derived from the Greek word *orgasmos,* means swollen organ, and of course does not depend upon sexual intercourse or even ejaculation.

Dear Dr. Kaufman:

I have a daughter 17 years of age who has a steady boyfriend. She has confided in me to the extent that she has a lot of conflict as to whether or not to have sexual intercourse. How do doctors advise adolescents in such a predicament?

Answer:

This can only be answered in general terms, since the specifics will necessarily vary with each individual situation. In probing into the background of the conflict of an adolescent girl (as posed in your question), the physician or counselor must consider several commonly encountered situations. One of the most common is where the girl is being pressured to have sexual relations to "prove her love." The male teenager's sex drive is mainly toward self-discovery, and his partner's wellbeing is usually not foremost in his mind. It is therefore not uncommon to find that, once coitus has taken place, the adolescent girl may confuse the sexual experience with a love relationship, or may have found the coital experience frightening, unsatisfying, and accompanied by much anxiety. Much depends upon her *emotional* readiness for sex.

It is important for the physician to provide a completely confidential and nonjudgmental setting in which the girl can vent her feelings. The fear of pregnancy and venereal disease should likewise be clarified, and means of prevention discussed.

Dear Dr. Kaufman:

Is direct stimulation of the clitoris essential for women to achieve orgasm?

Answer:

No. Even during intercourse it is difficult for the penis to make *direct* contact with the clitoris, and orgasm during coitus depends on the thrusting motion which creates friction between the lesser vaginal lips and the upper attachment to the clitoral hood.

Furthermore, some women can trigger orgasm by stimulation of other parts of their body, such as the ear canal, anus, or even through fantasy alone. Perhaps the ultimate proof is that when the clitoris is surgically removed (for some disease) orgasm is still possible.

Dear Dr. Kaufman:

I always need added lubrication to enjoy sex without discomfort, but this seems to be messy. What suggestions to you have?

Answer:

Whatever you apply should be put on the penis and not at the entrance to the vagina or in it. Far less will be required, with maximum benefit.

Dear Dr. Kaufman:

I notice that I am more sexually responsive before my menstrual periods. Is this common?

Answer:

Yes. Many women feel a definite increase in both sex drive and response premenstrually. Probably this is due to pelvic congestion. It is essentially the same physiological mechanism that causes the breasts to become fuller and more sensitive before a period.

Dear Dr. Kaufman:

Is it true the one can tell when a woman is having an orgasm by noting that her nipples become erect at that time?

Answer:

According to the findings of Masters and Johnson, there is no particular breast reponse to the orgasmic phase of sex, though it is true that in the early excitement phase there is usually nipple erection. Also, the area surrounding the nipple becomes engorged before and during orgasm and when this engorgement decreases (after orgasm) the nipples appear to be relatively erect.

Dear Dr. Kaufman:

My husband seems more concerned about whether or not I have an orgasm than his own enjoyment. Is this a common preoccupation?

Answer:

Yes it is, and it is often motivated by basic doubts concerning male competence. If he is functioning adequately, he should be reassured that your orgasm is not his primary problem. Sometimes a woman will not have an orgasm but still experience pleasure. Emphasis should be on love and tenderness, and this need not always culminate in orgasm.

Dear Dr. Kaufman:

I don't understand how, in this day and age, scientists still cannot agree as to whether there are two separate orgasms for women, clitoral and vaginal. Can you comment?

Answer:

Some authorities still hold to the concept of an independent vaginal orgasm, claiming that it comes from involuntary vaginal contractions. However, physiological research has shown that similar contractions occur with clitoral stimulation alone.

The long-standing debate over the vaginal orgasm is probably more of an emotional than a purely physiological matter. It may have to do with how a woman thinks about having something enter her body and whether she welcomes or rejects it.

We do know that the clitoris apparently has no other function than being the seat of erotic sensations, there being very few nerve endings in the vagina.

Dear Dr. Kaufman:

In regard to so-called clitoral versus vaginal orgasm, do you in your own practice find any discrepancy between what women report to you and the Masters-Johnson findings?

Answer:

They are not actually contradictory. Masters and Johnson found that the underlying physiological responses to stimulation were the same whether the source of stimulation was clitoral or vaginal. What women report to me are their own perceptions of sexual response, and some do feel a difference. For example, some women said that direct manual stimulation of the clitoris was not exciting, while others reported the opposite, with no response to vaginal stimulation. It may be that vaginally oriented women have a greater need to feel fused with someone, and perhaps clitorally oriented women have a greater need for more sexual independence. These are only conjectures of course, but they are worth pondering.

In any event, judging from my own clinical experience, it seems to me that much needless distress can be caused by the dictum that all women must achieve orgasm only by penile penetration, if only because a great number of women might think themselves "abnormal" and seek therapy because they are experiencing a satisfying orgasm but it is "only clitoral."

Dear Dr. Kaufman:

I have been married for 18 years, and from what I have read I can't help but feel that there is something to be said for the fact that monogamy lacks a certain variety that would otherwise come from sexual experiences with more than one individual. I would be interested in knowing your thoughts about this.

Answer:

Although the popular saying is "variety is the very spice of life" (written by William Cowper some two centuries ago), the more basic question is whether that variety can be achieved within marriage or must be looked for outside of marriage.

I would say that it all depends on how good a marital choice was made in the first place. If it was a good choice, we are not likely to want to hurt the partner in any way. For such marriages, familiarity may be said to breed content.

For others, adultery is a way of life—not so much because of the monotony of monogamy, but because the choice of marital partner was poor to begin with and there are very basic dissatisfactions and a gnawing feeling that things could be, and should be better.

Dear Dr. Kaufman:

I am 20 years old and just recently married. My problem is that I can't seem to have sexual relations with my husband, though we have tried several times. Apparently my pelvic region is overly small.

Answer:

One of the reasons a premarital physical examination is so important is that many anatomical and emotional blocks to sexual relations can be explored, detected, and corrected before the marriage night. Your problem may simply be that you are virginal—that is, the entrance to the vagina is too small for adequate penetration. A simple examination will disclose this. Gentle, gradual self-stretching will correct it.

Occasionally the difficulty is not anatomical at all, but emotional. That is, there is no actual narrowing at the vaginal entrance, but the woman is so tense and apprehensive that her vaginal muscles contract involuntarily and constrict the opening, preventing sexual penetration. This is called vaginismus, and requires careful explanation and reassurance by a physician skilled in the management of such psychosexual problems. Sometimes psychotherapy is also required.

Dear Dr. Kaufman:

We have been married a few weeks and no matter how hard we try, my hymen will not break. Please tell me what I can do.

Answer:

A medical examination will reveal such anatomic obstacles to intercourse as an intact, unyielding hymen, and the doctor can decide on the best remedy. Many women are afraid to see a doctor because they think he must painfully "break" the hymen. Not so. If examination discloses a narrow hymenal opening, the woman can be instructed to dilate herself very gradually, and therefore without much discomfort, using her own fingers or special vaginal dilators as a wedge. The hymenal ring is circular and, unlike a rubber band, it does not revert to its former size if stretched.

Dear Dr. Kaufman:

I have heard that women can improve sexual satisfaction by contracting certain pelvic muscles during intercourse. Can you explain what this is all about?

Answer:

In recent years there has been a good deal of discussion about one aspect of female sexual response sometimes called the "Exercise"—which is an awareness of, and the ability to squeeze, a pelvic muscle called the pubococcygeus. The contraction and good tone of this muscle can help stimulate deep nerve endings just beyond the vaginal walls during intercourse, and this can contribute to sexual satisfaction. This same muscle contracts spasmodically and involuntarily during female orgasm.

Some women can contract the muscle deliberately, once they know it exists; others need specific instruction. There are several ways in which a woman can identify the pubococcygeus, but the easiest is simply to interrupt the urinary flow. Actually, exercises for these muscles were originally devised for the relief of distressing urinary leakage in women whose pelvic muscles were too relaxed.

It should be added that many women who are made aware of this muscle do report increased sexual pleasure, but the results are by no means uniform or consistent. Because a woman's orgasm is so intimately bound to her emotions, it is not surprising that many women with excellently developed pelvic muscles prove to be sexually unresponsive, whereas others can have a high degree of orgastic response even with marked pelvic relaxations.

Dear Dr. Kaufman:

Is it true that many women before menopause sublimate their sexual needs through various nonsexual activities, but suddenly demand frequent intercourse when they reach menopause? Would not such new and unexpected demands on their sexual participation jolt some husbands out of their possibly comfortable adjustment?

Answer:

What you say is certainly sometimes true. Menopause happens to be a stark reminder to any woman that she is getting older, possibly less attractive. In our present-day, youth-oriented culture this is a depressing thought. The reaction to such feelings can either take the form of further sexual inhibition or, as in the example you cited, there may be an attempt to reinstate "youthful" sexual vigor by an almost compulsive wish for frequent sexual intercourse. It is the same sort of anxiety that often brings a middle-aged woman who has just missed her first period to the doctor "worried" about pregnancy. Although she anticipates and receives reassurance (after examination) that the verdict is menopause, there is nevertheless an understandable nostalgic reminiscence of years gone by, when the fear of "getting caught" was very real.

In my own clinical experience, I have found that these subtle emotional feelings play a much greater role than the apparently more obvious and frequently cited explanations of postmenopausal sexual surge—namely, freedom from contraceptive needs.

Dear Dr. Kaufman:

Could you comment on the sex drive according to age, in both the male and female?

Answer:

In general, males are highly sexual during youth, reach their peak in the late teens or early twenties, then gradually decline thereafter. Women are, by comparison, not as intensely sexually oriented during youth but slowly become so, reaching their erotic peak in middle age, declining slowly afterward.

Some wit has plotted a graph indicating the rising ascent of female response and the slow decline of male response, then showing how the two graphs cross at about the age 34, for about an hour!

Dear Dr. Kaufman:

I am 49, still have regular periods, but have noticed that my sexual urges have diminished considerably in the last year or so. Could this be due to approaching menopause?

Answer:

No. Many people (men, as well as women) still have the mistaken notion that menopause brings with it a loss of sexual drive. Actually, menopause results in the loss of menstrual periods and reproductive function, but has no *direct* bearing on libido. Sexual desires and responses are emotionally governed, at any age.

Dear Dr. Kaufman:

Do you ever recommend sex manuals for patients who are having problems with their sex life?

Answer:

Not often, because there is a tendency for the "book" to become another "dictator" to their activities, increasing their anxieties and self-consciousness. However, reading a book together can sometimes open channels of communication between the partners. When such communication is obviously difficult, I often say to the couple: "Why don't you write your *own* book?"

Dear Dr. Kaufman:

When I recently consulted my family doctor about the fact that I have very little desire for sex, he kind of shrugged it off. Whom can I talk to about this if not my family physician?

Answer:

Ideally, you should be able to communicate such feelings directly to your husband, especially since the desire for sex is very much dependent upon one's interpersonal relationship. Assuming that you cannot, and do seek outside help, it is admittedly often difficult to obtain a sympathetic ear.

I'm reminded of a patient who had a similar complaint—an attractive young woman in her twenties. She mentioned that she had no desire for sex and had previously consulted another doctor, her family physician, who happened to be in his seventies. When I asked her why she hadn't gone back to him, she answered, "I told him my problem, that I had no desire for sex, and all he said was, 'Neither do I!' "

Because so many doctors are reluctant to discuss sexual problems, or do not have the time, it has fallen largely into the realm of the gynecologist and obstetrician. There are also other areas of help: a psychologist, psychiatrist, a member of the American Association of Marriage Counselors, and various sex therapy teams, according to the specific problem.

Dear Dr. Kaufman:

I have read several marriage and sex manuals, most of which depict the sexual act in a stereotyped way. The chief role of the male is to satisfy his partner, and apparently the worst thing that can happen is for him to reach orgasm before she is "fulfilled." Is this not difficult advice to follow?

Answer:

It certainly is. In general, I have reservations about the kind of sexual activity advised as ideal by many sex manuals. In fact, I noted that in one such book, the following advice is given for the couple where the male apparently reaches a climax at an inopportune moment:

"Before intercourse, the wife places at the bedside a bowl of crushed ice or a handful of cracked ice wrapped in a wet towel. Both partners strip and enjoy sex in any face-to-face posture, with the husband on top. As the husband starts his final surge to climax, the wife picks up a handful of crushed ice or the cold towel. Just as the paroxysms of orgasm start, she jams the ice cold poultice against her husband's crotch and keeps it there throughout the conclusion."

Many manuals are, to a lesser extent, restrictive. In my opinion, people should not have to restrain, control, and suppress their emotions and impulses in order to achieve sexual satisfaction.

Dear Dr. Kaufman:

Just how important is technical expertise in sex? For example, does the failure to achieve simultaneous orgasm necessarily reflect an inadequate or incomplete sexual relationship?

Answer:

Technique is important only to the extent that it enables a couple to give and receive pleasure. Simultaneous orgasm is difficult to achieve and should certainly not be the "goal."

Dear Dr. Kaufman:

I wonder what you think about these marriage manuals that constantly advise women to buy slinky negligees and avoid walking around in hair curlers.

Answer:

I think such advice is really superfluous for any woman who likes her man. For those who don't, the advice will be ignored.

Dear Dr. Kaufman:

Some say that sexual conflict is the chief *cause* of marital discord, and others say it is the *result* of a poor marriage. I would be interested in knowing your opinion. I would also like to know how you would describe a "good" sexual relationship.

Answer:

I would say that sexual conflict is both cause *and* effect, and often an accompaniment to general marital disharmony.

A good sexual relationship does not require volumes of sex manuals for description. The basic prerequisite is that the couple not only love each other but like each other. Everything else follows. Sometimes they will be close and affectionate, other times solemnly passionate, and still other times utterly frivolous or play-acting. There is no reluctance, on occasion, to have intercourse as a plain bodily need, with no romanticism at all. The couple is uninhibited, and happy with each other.

Such well adjusted couples accept the fact that at any given moment their desire for sex is never exactly equal, and they consider this just as natural as their differing appetites at a restaurant. However, since sex is a shared experience, they are happy to compromise. This does not mean that a man doesn't care if his wife seems not in the mood on occasion; of course he cares, and he may dislike it. He may equally dislike having to respond if *he* is not in the mood. But in a good marriage such episodes are simply not going to throw either one of them, and they are not taken seriously.

Dear Dr. Kaufman:

My husband and I are in conflict. He happens to enjoy cunnilingus as a prelude to intercourse, while I personally do not like this method of foreplay. We have no other sexual difficulties. Please advise.

Answer:

The *easiest* advice is simply to say that since oral-genital contact is obviously not mutually desired, forget it. However, my clinical hunch is that the sexual difficulty you describe may reflect a broader and deeper problem in your interpersonal relationship. Not uncommonly, a couple is engaged in a kind of power struggle for control, and it would be of interest to explore how you deal with other aspects of your relationship—child rearing, money, leisure time, and so on. If there is evidence of additional battles for control, you would probably benefit by some sound marital counseling.

Dear Dr. Kaufman:

I have been married twelve years and have always been unable to reach a climax during intercourse, but always have a very satisfactory orgasm if my husband stimulates my clitoris some other way. The thing that disturbs me is that I think of this as "masturbation" and this bothers me. Is this a common problem?

Answer:

It's common, but I wouldn't necessarily call it a "problem." What you have been doing for twelve years is to mark each sexual experience as a failure or disappointment, instead of the actual pleasure you feel it to be. Instead of considering this to be masturbation, have you ever considered that when your husband does these things to you, he is *caressing* you in a very special way? It could make all the difference!

Dear Dr. Kaufman:

Do you find that people who harbor the idea that sex is sinful neglect to use birth control?

Answer:

Yes. Dislike, fear, or distaste of sex makes it harder to use birth control. Professional help is usually required, not so much for birth control as for the exploration of sexual hang-ups.

I also believe that the inclusion of sex in the school curriculum would be a helpful step toward open discussion of one of the most important of human functions. However, such teaching should be by teachers who are themselves knowledgeable and open-minded, not like the one in the cartoon who addressed her class of youngsters by saying, "I am required to teach you about sex, reproduction, and other disgusting filth."

Dear Dr. Kaufman:

We have been married 23 years and it's been stormy all the way. Trouble is, we both have strong personalities and don't see eye to eye on most things, whether it be sex, the children (though they're pretty much on their own now), or how we should spend our leisure time. It seems to me that my husband has become more stubborn in recent years. Anyway, our sex life has begun to deteriorate and I'm just concerned that we might not make it to our 25th anniversary. I know you probably need more details, but wondered if you have any suggestions off the top?

Answer:

I would bet that you do reach your golden anniversary. There are many marital relationships that have been aptly described as the "durable, incompatible marriage." On the surface, the marriage seems ready to collapse from the very first year, yet the couple sticks together for as many years as you have. Apparently there is something in the personality makeup in both of you that actually requires the disharmony you describe. A very skilled professional counselor would be needed to untangle the kind of set pattern you have both developed.

Dear Dr. Kaufman:

I know that there are no true aphrodisiac foods, but has anyone ever mentioned music? I find that certain kinds of music and rhythms can be sexually very stimulating.

Answer:

It's true, you don't hear much about music as a sexual stimulant, probably because it would depend very much on one's individual reaction. However, you may recall the famous painting (used in perfume advertisements) showing a male violinist embracing a female pianist. It is supposed to illustrate the climactic moment of Tolstoy's moralistic novel *The Kreutzer Sonata.* The title refers to Beethoven's Sonata for violin and piano, dedicated to Rodolphe Kreutzer. According to the story, the last, syncopated movement of this sonata possessed such aphrodisiac powers that it drove the players (a married woman and a male violinist) into an uncontrollable, illicit love affair. (Before rushing to your record player let me just add that I think the second movement is much more sensuous!)

Dear Dr. Kaufman:

What is a wet dream? My boyfriend has never had one so he can't explain it. Do girls get it too?

Answer:

It is interesting that in this day and age, with the numerous sexual outlets available to young people, wet dreams are relatively uncommon. Known as nocturnal emissions, such dreams have an erotic element which culminate in actual orgasm. Girls can certainly have dreams ending in orgasm, but since there is no fluid discharge such dreams will not be "wet."

Dear Dr. Kaufman:

If a man and woman have intercourse the night before she went to the doctor for an examination, could he tell that she had had intercourse the night before?

Answer:

It is possible that the doctor could, if he specifically examines the secretions from the cervix under the microscope for the presence of sperm. Sperm can often be detected in this area, even after 24-48 hours, if it happens to be a "favorable" time of the cycle—that is, near ovulation.

Dear Dr. Kaufman:

I wondered what your opinion is of self-help groups which urge self-examination of one's vagina and cervix?

Answer:

I think it's natural that women are interested in their own bodies. They want to know more about its structure. Gynecologists try to do just that when teaching a woman what to feel for when inserting a diaphragm. I see no harm in a woman's looking at her cervix with a plastic speculum and mirror. The obvious limitation of self-examination is that it is understandably difficult for a woman to interpret what she sees, if it is at all out of the ordinary, without adequate medical background.

Dear Dr. Kaufman:

I read somewhere that there was a book by a doctor describing how sex can keep you slim. How is that possible? (I am an overweight lady of 33.)

Answer:

It's an intriguing thought. Actually, I don't know of any exact scientific studies which measure the precise energy expenditure for sexual activity (obviously it would be different under different circumstances). Those studies in which researchers have extrapolated heart rate responses during sex mention a total energy output of about 75 calories, similar to climbing one or two flights of stairs. One observer calculated that if a person had sexual relations every day for a full year (maintaining everything else constant), he or she would reduce body weight by only six to eight pounds.

NINE

The Breasts

Dear Dr. Kaufman:

Is the size of a woman's breasts related to her sexual drive?

Answer:

No. Sexual drives are cerebral in origin, and the size of the breasts is unrelated.

Dear Dr. Kaufman:

What is the best way for a woman to examine her own breasts?

Answer:

Lie down and put one hand behind your head. With the other hand, fingers flattened, feel the opposite breast gently, and then the armpit. The time to do this is right after your menstrual period when the breasts are softest. Doing it each month enables you to become familiar with your breasts and to detect changes (such as a lump). Use the opposite hand to examine the opposite breast, in the same way. Be sure to continue these checkups once a month, even after menopause, for the rest of your life. It is important to see your physician if you discover a lump or thickening.

Dear Dr. Kaufman:

I am 37, have five children, but have a very small bust. I have been working very hard at exercises and I eat a good dairy diet, but nothing happens. I want to go to a plastic surgeon, but my husband won't let me. Can something be done for me?

Answer:

Apparently your husband likes you just the way you are, and that's the important thing. Diet and exercise are rather ineffectual, as you have already found. Plastic surgery is the only sure way of changing your bust size, but the results of surgery are not always ideal in terms of the way the breast feels to the touch, even though the bust may look better. Why not go along with your husband?

Dear Dr. Kaufman:

My 18-year-old daughter insists on going without a bra. Can this be medically harmful?

Answer:

To my knowledge, going without a bra presents no known harm for well supported breasts, particularly in a young lady.

Dear Dr. Kaufman:

I am one of five daughters. My mother and two of my sisters have well developed breasts. But three of us (including myself) never developed much of a bosom. Can anything be done by injection to solve our problem?

Answer:

If you mean injection into the breast, the answer is no. Injection of a foreign substance, such as silicone, directly into the breast is dangerous and legally prohibited. However, the injection of female hormones into the arm, or the ingestion of such hormones as are contained in birth control pills, do have an effect upon the breasts. They become larger, but only because of fluid retention; there is actually no increased breast tissue. Consequently, the effect is transient and disappears when such hormone therapy ceases. The only safe way to increase breast size permanently is by competent plastic surgery.

Dear Dr. Kaufman:

Please explain what determines the size of one's breasts. I always thought it was in proportion to body size. I have a friend who measures 42-26-37. The reason I know her measurements is because she asked me to make some clothes for her.

Answer:

Like other physical features, breast size is determined largely by heredity. The initial impetus to growth is hormonally governed. Of course, a person's weight also plays a role, with the breasts receiving their fair share of an increase in fat. Those women who have been endowed with a large amount of glandular breast tissue will seem relatively top-heavy.

Dear Dr. Kaufman:

I suffer pains in my breasts and am told I might have cystic mastitis. Please explain what that is and what can be done.

Answer:

Cystic mastitis is a condition in which a portion or portions of the breast have a tendency toward multiple glandular cysts. The filling of these cysts with fluid and their distention cause pain. Estrogenic hormone tends to aggravate the condition; progesterone tends to alleviate it. The discomfort is also lessened by anything that helps drive out excess body fluid, such as a diuretic. Some doctors give large doses of vitamin B complex as it may help the liver deactivate estrogen.

Dear Dr. Kaufman:

I am 23 and have a problem that has worried me since age 16. One of my breasts is considerably larger than the other. My husband doesn't seem to mind, but he tells me that if I lose 25 pounds (I am quite heavy) this problem will disappear. I have my doubts. What do you think?

Answer:

Seldom does any woman have breasts exactly the same size, but I gather that in your case the difference is significant. Losing weight (a good idea, in any event) will decrease the size of both your breasts, though they may remain disproportionate. Since your husband doesn't mind, why not just diet and see what happens? The only alternatives are wearing a special bra or plastic surgery, the latter being an expensive procedure.

Dear Dr. Kaufman:

My daughter is 15. She has been menstruating for two years, but her breasts are still rather small. Is this abnormal? Can anything be done?

Answer:

The fact that your daughter has been menstruating for two years indicates that she does not lack estrogenic hormonal stimulation. The degree to which breasts are stimulated to grow varies with the individual and her particular genetic endowment. Her breast development should not be considered "abnormal."

TEN

Venereal Disease

Dear Dr. Kaufman:

I am 23 years old and must admit to sexual contacts with many men. I worry about venereal disease, and several doctors I have gone to have taken tests for gonorrhea. One took a culture from the cervix, another from the cervix and bladder opening. I wonder whether there is any standard diagnostic procedures that could ease my anxiety.

Answer:

The areas from which the gonorrheal organism can be cultured include the cervix, the urethra, the rectum, and even the throat. Eighty per cent of women who have gonorrhea do not show any symptoms of the disease. Sometimes their disease is recognized only after more serious complications develop. The other problem with VD testing is that even if all areas tested are negative on one occasion, the woman can develop gonorrhea (or syphilis) the very next day through another contact; retesting is required each time.

A properly collected *culture* (particularly from the cer-

vix) will detect the disorder in about 9 cases out of 10. A smear alone will detect gonorrhea in only about 5 out of 10 infected women.

Dear Dr. Kaufman:

What causes syphilis?

Answer:

A spiral-shaped organism called a spirochete. It is the most deadly of venereal diseases. The spirochete cannot be seen with an ordinary microscope, but only under a special dark-field microscope which few physicians have. However, such dark-field services are available in most large cities.

There are also standardized blood tests (serology) to alert the physician that a syphilitic infection may be present.

Dear Dr. Kaufman:

If a person has venereal disease, would every sexual contact result in an infection to the partner?

Answer:

No. Neither syphilis nor gonorrhea is 100 per cent infectious. On the average, one person will become infected out of every four who have intercourse with someone who has infectious syphilis. For gonorrhea the figures are one in three for sexual contact with a person who has an acute case, and one in twelve for contact with a chronic case (where the germs are relatively sparse).

For a person to contract syphilis, the spirochete must penetrate the mucous membrane. Just touching a syphilitic sore with your hand would probably not result in infection. Contact would have to be made with mucous membrane, which could be the mouth, vagina, penis, and so on.

Dear Dr. Kaufman:

Which disease—syphilis or gonorrhea—goes back further in history?

Answer:

Gonorrhea is considered the older of these venereal diseases. It was rather well described in 2,637 B.C. by the Chinese Emperor Hoang-Ti, as an inflammation of the urethra caused by contact of the penis with some peculiar matter produced by a woman's genitals.

Gonorrhea was also known to the ancient Hebrews. About 1,500 B.C. Moses (in Leviticus 15) spoke of an infectious discharge and suggested sanitary regulations. The disease was also known to the ancient Greeks and Romans, and was well described by Hippocrates about 460 B.C.

The actual name "gonorrhea" was given by the Greek physician, Galen, who practiced in Rome. However, it was not until 1879 that Neisser isolated the germ causing this disease, and he called it the "gonococcus." It is today still known also as "Neisserian" infection.

At the present time, gonorrhea is the most prevalent of the venereal diseases throughout the world. In the United States alone, there are about 1½ million new cases a year. There are about 20 cases of gonorrhea for every case of syphilis.

Dear Dr. Kaufman:

What is the best way to prevent venereal disease?

Answer:

Since venereal disease is a sexually transmitted disease, the best preventive is, of course, avoidance of sexual contact where there is a possibility of such transmission. In this regard, it might be pointed out that, among the various methods of contraception, the condom can protect simultaneously against pregnancy and venereal disease in the majority of cases.

Many experts are advising the return to an overlooked technique of control, namely, plain soap and water. They point out that if sexual partners washed or douched genital areas before and after contact (or at least after), the risk of infection would be expected to decrease significantly. The mechanical action of washing removes some of the germs, and the soapy fluid aids in killing many more. It is of interest that in France, where the bidet is commonly used, the incidence of gonorrhea is relatively low.

Dear Dr. Kaufman:

Does a person have immunity to VD after having had it?

Answer:

No, a person can be re-infected again and again.

Dear Dr. Kaufman:

Are there venereal diseases other than syphilis and gonorrhea?

Answer:

Yes. Other sexually transmitted (venereal) diseases include genital herpes (a virus), trichomonas (a harmless parasitic infection), pubic lice (crabs), and much rarer diseases known as chancroid and lymphogranuloma venereum.

Dear Dr. Kaufman:

When is the most infectious time for spreading syphilis?

Answer:

Syphilis is spread in two brief periods of time: when the person is in the primary stage, which may last for a week or two, and when the person is in the secondary stage. In contrast, gonorrhea may be infectious for a much longer time—for many months rather than weeks.

Dear Dr. Kaufman:

Can a person become infected with syphilis and gonorrhea at the same time?

Answer:

Yes. One can also catch either disease many times.

Dear Dr. Kaufman:

I have heard that gonorrhea can occur in children. How is this possible without sexual contact?

Answer:

Gonorrheal infection can be transmitted to a small child by any intimate contact with an infected person. The newborn infant passing through its infected mother's birth canal can develop a gonorrheal eye infection. The small child can, of course, contract gonorrhea through direct sexual contact, whether heterosexual or homosexual.

Opinions vary as to whether gonorrheal infection can be transmitted to small children by *indirect*, non-sexual contact. Many believe this may occur under special conditions of severe overcrowding, shared sleeping facilities, poor personal hygiene, and of course high incidence of gonorrhea among the adults.

The gonorrheal organism is very delicate, and succumbs to the effect of drying within an hour or two. However, it may remain viable for short periods of time outside the body if it is in a moist environment.

Dear Dr. Kaufman:

Will a baby be born with syphilis if the mother is infected?

Answer:

If the mother receives treatment during the first four months of pregnancy, the baby will escape infection. If not, the disease may be transmitted to the baby, causing deformity or stillbirth.

Dear Dr. Kaufman:

What are the early and late symptoms and signs of syphilis?

Answer:

The first sign of infection is a painless sore, at the point where the germ has entered the body. It appears between two to six weeks after exposure and disappears without treatment, but this only means that the disease has gone deeper into the body.

The second stage of syphilis, which can start anywhere between two to six months after the initial sore, can include skin rashes over all or part of the body, patchy baldness, sore throat, fever, and headaches. But even these signs will disappear without treatment. However, the disease remains in the body (without treatment), and can eventually cause nervous system crippling, insanity, heart disease, and death.

Dear Dr. Kaufman:

What are the main symptoms of gonorrhea?

Answer:

In men, the main symptoms are a painful, burning sensation when urinating, and a discharge of pus from the penis. In women, about 80 per cent show no attention-drawing symptoms. Sometimes there is a pus-like discharge and slight burning on urination that occurs from 3 days to 3 weeks following exposure. But these are early symptoms and signs. Later, there may be ascending infection into the Fallopian tubes, with resulting abdominal pains, fever, and often sterility. Ascending infection in men can also lead to inflammation of the testicular area with subsequent sterility. In both men and women, other systemic complications of gonorrhea include arthritis, blindness, heart trouble, and death.

Dear Dr. Kaufman:

One hears a lot about the rising rate of venereal disease. What effect will this have on the fertility of those involved?

Answer:

Without doubt, an adverse effect. The commonest venereal disease, gonorrhea, can cause permanent sterility in both male and female victims unless treated promptly and adequately. Females are especially vulnerable since early signs and symptoms in women are often minimal or go completely unnoticed. Unnoticed, that is, in the early stage, but definitely noticed if and when the infection spreads to the delicate Fallopian tubes. It is in this region that destructive damage so often results in sterility.

Dear Dr. Kaufman:

Is rectal gonorrhea possible in a woman if she has not engaged in anal coitus?

Answer:

Yes, although anal coitus is the most likely way of acquiring it. Transmission of the gonorrheal germ to the rectum may occur by spread from the vagina.

Dear Dr. Kaufman:

Is it true that the organism causing syphilis is more resistant to penicillin today than it was years ago?

Answer:

No. There is no evidence that it is more resistant today. However, there are strains of *gonorrhea* that are significantly more resistant to penicillin today, compared with 10 or 20 years ago.

Dear Dr. Kaufman:

A doctor recently took a smear from my throat and said that I had gonorrhea of that region. I do not see how this is possible in my particular case. Could this be a laboratory error?

Answer:

A "positive" *smear* from the pharynx is not necessarily indicative of gonorrheal infection. Epidemiological studies have shown that a certain percentage of the population are carriers of *meningococci,* and these smears resemble those of gonorrhea and can be confused with the disease. Gonorrhea of the pharynx cannot be established with certainty without a positive *culture.*

Dear Dr. Kaufman:

Can gonorrhea of the throat be contracted by either kissing or cunnilingus?

Answer:

No. In almost every case where there is a gonorrheal pharyngitis (as proven by culture), the infection has been by fellatio. Gonorrheal pharyngitis apparently does not occur from cunnilingus or kissing. Interestingly, the gonorrheal organism has not been isolated from the mouth cavity, but only from the pharynx and tonsilar area. In such cases, the organism can usually be found also in the cervix, urethra or rectum.

ELEVEN

Female Troubles

Dear Dr. Kaufman:

Can you discuss painful menstrual periods? I am a school teacher and find that a great many of my high school girls complain of this affliction and are often absent for a day or more each month.

Answer:

Painful menstruation, known as dysmenorrhea, is a very common problem, particularly among younger women, although no age group is exempt during the childbearing years. Severity of symptoms varies from an hour or two ot discomfort to incapacitating pains for several days. A complete history and physical examination are essential.

Physical causes include a marked narrowing of the cervix, which responds favorably to simple dilatation. Or, the womb may be severely tipped and immobile due to chronic pelvic infection.

Another physical cause of increasingly painful periods is

known as endometriosis, a condition in which bits of tissue usually found only in the lining of the womb are present outside the womb–on the ovary or intestines, for example. These bits of misplaced lining cells can react during each menstrual period by bleeding, causing pain and even scarring of surrounding tissues. A common form of treatment is by high doses of estrogen and progesterone to produce what is known as a "false pregnancy," since the menstrual periods are completely suppressed; with such treatment the endometriosis begins literally to melt away.

In most cases of dysmenorrhea, however, no physical cause is found. There may also be a large emotional component.

Interestingly, women who do not ovulate rarely have painful periods. (This does not mean that women with painless periods have an ovulation problem.) Thus, suppressing ovulation, as with birth control pills, eliminates the pain.

Many respond to much simpler therapy, such as small doses of male hormone for a few days preceding ovulation, which does not interfere with ovulation at all.

Most physicians treat dysmenorrhea with simple analgesics, antispasmodics, and reassurance, often with good results.

Dear Dr. Kaufman:

Why is it that women who have suffered for years with painful menstruation are "cured" after they have had a baby? It has happened to me as well as to many of my friends. Can this "cure" be expected to last for life?

Answer:

Most cases of painful menstruation are associated with strong uterine contractions combined with a relative narrowing of the cervical canal. Very often just stretching the cervix with dilators (an office procedure) will relieve a woman of painful menstruation for months. Obviously, there is no better stretching than childbirth, which accounts for the "cure." In addition, a uterus that has contained a pregnancy is generally less prone to undergo contractions during each period, hence less pain.

Dear Dr. Kaufman:

I know that fear or emotional stress can cause a woman to miss her period, but I don't understand how this actually comes about. Please explain.

Answer:

The easiest explanation is to look at menstruation as an interplay of certain glands—the ovaries, pituitary, adrenals, and thyroid. These glands are all influenced by the "seat of the emotions," or midbrain (*hypothalamus*). If, for example, the hypothalamus is upset by fear or emotional stress, the whole mechanism of glandular interaction is interfered with, and the result may well be a missed or delayed period.

Dear Dr. Kaufman:

I have heard of a pill which is supposed to bring on a period within four days if a woman is "late." Could you describe how this works? Is this the same as the "morning after" pill?

Answer:

The pills you are referring to can be either progesterone alone, or a combination of estrogen and progesterone—in either case given for several days. A menstrual flow is likely to start within a few days, *but only if there is no pregnancy.*

Such pills will not abort an established pregnancy. The medication is completely different from so-called "morning after" medication which, of course, is used within a few days after exposure and not when one is already "late."

Dear Dr. Kaufman:

My niece who is 21 needs help. Two years ago, on her own, she went on a diet and lost a lot of weight even though she was not too fat. Shortly afterward her periods stopped, and one doctor doubted that she could have any children. She is very worried. So am I. Can you comment?

Answer:

A "crash" diet with sudden loss of a lot of weight can interfere with hormonal function and cause menstrual periods to stop altogether. Although such a condition often stubbornly resists medical therapy, it is usually self-limiting, meaning that eventually the periods return spontaneously. In some cases, this takes a few years. Luckily, your niece is still young and the chances are that, given enough time, her fertility will return spontaneously.

Dear Dr. Kaufman:

My 15-year-old daughter is five foot three and weighs almost 160 pounds. Her periods, which began when she was 12, have become irregular. I have always encouraged her to eat a proper diet, but perhaps I overdid it. How can I get her to lose some weight now? She refuses to listen to my advice.

Answer:

Many studies have shown that eating disorders can be traced to early family influences. Too many youngsters are told to clean their plate; actually, if the youngster's weight is normal, he or she should be told simply to eat till filled, then stop. Unfortunately, in some unstable home surroundings, food becomes a substitute for love and security.

I doubt whether your advice to eat less *now* will be heeded. Your best bet is to have your family doctor take over this responsibility. And don't be concerned about her irregular periods during these adolescent years.

Dear Dr. Kaufman:

I've heard that there are exercises that can help painful periods. Could you mention what specific exercise can be tried?

Answer:

There are several. One popular one is for the woman to turn her trunk to the left, then bend and touch her left foot with her right hand, attempting to reach around the other side of her left foot to touch the heel. This is repeated on the opposite side.

Another exercise is to stretch out flat on the floor on one's back with knees bent. The knees are then separated, keeping the feet on the floor near the buttocks. The lower end of the spine is then lifted off the floor. Repeat.

Still another is to lie on your back, arms at the sides, palms up. The knees are drawn up over the chest; slowly straighten the legs up. Now the knees are bent and the feet are placed flat on the floor as close to the buttocks as possible. Repeat.

Dear Dr. Kaufman:

I have been plagued by premenstrual tension for many years. I wonder if you could discuss this subject and tell me if anything can be done about it. Not only do I have a washed-out feeling, but I actually look "different" before my period, though otherwise I'm told I'm pretty.

Answer:

The term "premenstrual tension" was coined by Dr. Robert T. Frank in 1931. The syndrome is characterized by many symptoms and occurs commonly in at least three out of four women of childbearing age. The complaints may include restlessness, irritability, headache, insomnia, backache, fatigue, pelvic heaviness, breast engorgement, emotional outbursts, crying spells, anxiety, tremors, alterations in personality, transient weight gain, and swelling, especially of the fingers and ankles. Not all these signs and symptoms, of course, are present at one time or in every woman. While the pattern is fairly consistent for the individual woman, the severity of symptoms varies from one's cycle to another. The weight gain averages three to five pounds premenstrually, but may be even more.

Undoubtedly fluid retention plays a role in the cause of this very common and annoying affliction. Yet the exact mechanism of the whole syndrome remains obscure. Common theories include an excess of estrogen, a relative decrease in progesterone, an imbalance of the sex hormones, emotional factors, and many other explanations.

Treatment is individualized: diuretics, tranquilizers, androgens, progesterones, low salt intake, vitamin B complex, and pills (such as birth control pills) to prevent ovulation are used as aids. Since symptoms vary from month to month it is often not possible to ascribe improvements specifically to the medication given. However, most women suffering from premenstrual tension can definitely be helped by the use of one or more of the measures mentioned.

Dear Dr. Kaufman:

I have been troubled by premenstrual depression, which has been greatly helped by diuretics. However, I get very weak when I take the pills. Is there a reason?

Answer:

Diuretics, or "water pills" as they are commonly called, can cause a depletion of important body minerals, chiefly potassium. This, in turn, can cause the symptoms of lassitude that you describe. However, it is relatively easy to counteract this effect by purposely eating foods rich in potassium. Excellent sources are oranges, bananas, dried apricots and figs. Other sources of potassium are meats, liver, fish, asparagus, beets, and broccoli; but remember that a lot of potassium is lost when foods are refined or when cooking water is poured down the drain. Therefore the fruits mentioned are more reliable sources.

Dear Dr. Kaufman:

Every month, about two weeks before my period, I get severe abdominal pains lasting for a day or two. I am told that this is due to the release of an egg each month. Can anything be done to stop this recurring discomfort? How common is it?

Answer:

About 25 per cent of all women of childbearing age experience some degree of mid-month discomfort due to ovulation. Such pain is less common in women in their forties, when ovulation begins to falter.

Typically, there is gradual onset of pain which is crampy and located in the lower abdomen. Sometimes the pain is confined to one side and, if severe, may be confused with other conditions such as appendicitis, especially if there is any nausea.

Mid-month pain may be accompanied by slight staining and nervous tension, and the onset of the following menstrual period is almost exactly two weeks after the onset of the pain.

Although related to impending or recent ovulation, the exact cause of the pain is obscure. In terms of treatment, a complete history and physical examination are important. When symptoms are mild, discussion and reassurance often suffice. Sometimes an analgesic may be needed for a day or two. In severe, recurrent cases, such as yours, temporary inhibition of ovulation with hormones usually prevents the pain completely.

Dear Dr. Kaufman:

What can be done to stop the growth of a female teenager who is embarrassingly tall for her age?

Answer:

The use of estrogen could be considered, but only after very careful evaluation by an endocrinologist.

Estrogen controls bone growth by normally closing bony ends, preventing further growth. The reason men are generally taller than women is that the "bone closing" effect of the female sex hormone estrogen is more marked than that of the male sex hormone, testosterone.

Dear Dr. Kaufman:

I am 22 years old and considered attractive. When I comb my hair, however, it seems that a good deal of it is left on the comb, and this concerns me. Can this be caused by lack of hormones?

Answer:

The growth and loss of hair is very complex. When scalp hair comes out, many persons confuse the knob at the end as the root. However, the knob is really the part of the shaft that fits into the root follicle. It regenerates and is therefore replaceable.

Hair follicles have a built-in rhythm of activity that results in a periodic moulting of old hair (resting phase) and growth of new. Hormones are just one controlling factor in the growth of hair. The hair you see on your comb represents mainly the hair in the resting phase.

Lack of the thyroid hormone, controlled in turn by the pituitary, is characterized by poor hair growth. The loss of hair commonly observed after the birth of a baby is undoubtedly related to a hormonal shift. Other important factors related to hair growth and loss are heredity, nutrition, and certain diseases.

Dear Dr. Kaufman:

Is it true that girls begin to menstruate and mature physically at an earlier age nowadays than years ago? If so what would account for this earlier sexual development and earlier menses?

Answer:

Yes, it's true. About a century ago the average age of first menses was about 17. Now it's down to 13 and still dropping. The reasons are not clear.

It's interesting that identical twins usually tend to begin menstruation within one or two months of each other, suggesting a hereditary factor. It is also of interest that the age at which menstruation finally ceases (menopause) has gotten progressively later, suggesting that the pituitary is somehow involved in the genesis of both trends.

Dear Dr. Kaufman:

I am almost 16 years old but have not yet menstruated. Is this abnormal?

Answer:

Ninety-five per cent of adolescents will have begun to menstruate by age 16. Occasionally the onset is not until age 17 or even 18, but if menses have not yet occurred by that age, an examination is warranted.

Irrespective of whether the onset of menstruation occurs at 10 or at 16, there is a sequence of anatomic events that normally takes place in all girls just before menses begin. First, breast budding appears, followed by the appearance of pubic and axillary hair, and finally by a spurt in height. If one sees such signs in progress, one can assume that menses will follow. However, if the girl is short, does not have any development of breasts, and does not have pubic hair, one must suspect a glandular deficiency.

Dear Dr. Kaufman:

I have heard that some girls have a completely closed hymen. How are they able to menstruate if this is so?

Answer:

They can't. When the hymen is completely closed, the monthly menstrual flow is actually blocked; it accumulates in the vagina, producing distention and severe monthly cramps, but without any signs of bleeding.

When the diagnosis is delayed, the backup may build up into the uterus and tubes to such an extent that it appears as a mass in the lower abdomen. In such cases there may be inflammation of the tubes, with consequent sterility.

Usually the condition is recognized long before this stage is reached, and is completely relieved by surgical incision of the hymen. When this is done, the old, dammed-up menstrual blood comes out.

Dear Dr. Kaufman:

Is it safe to use tampons as soon as one begins menstruating as an adolescent?

Answer:

A girl can begin using tampons at any time. Tense muscles or a small vaginal opening (hymen) may make insertion more difficult the first few times but usually there is enough room, especially if a little lubricant is used initially. A tampon does not "block" the flow of blood, but merely absorbs it.

Dear Dr. Kaufman:

Does estrogen have any therapeutic benefits other than for menopausal symtpoms?

Answer:

Estrogens have many therapeutic uses: for the control of acne, for the treatment of painful periods, excessive hairiness, poor breast development, inhibition of lactation, certain vaginal inflammations, and some types of infertility problems with hormonal imbalance. Estrogen has also been helpful in treating the pain of osteoporosis, for the management of the growth of the excessively tall girl, to control some types of abnormal uterine bleeding, to increase the quantity of cervical mucus, and even as a therapeutic means of treating breast cancer postoperatively in postmenopausal women who are more than five years past menopause. Preventively, estrogen is also the chief ingredient of most contraceptive pills.

Dear Dr. Kaufman:

Is it true that women are the biologically superior sex?

Answer:

No question about it. And it starts at conception. Although more males are conceived than females, more miscarriages and stillbirths happen to males. In twin pregnancies, if a male and female are competing for space, survival is decidedly higher among females. Congenital anomalies are more common among males. Later in life, coronary disease, the prime killer, is much more common in men. Actuarial statistics show that a female's life expectancy is 75 at birth. A man, however, has to survive to age 50 in order to gain the same expectancy.

Dear Dr. Kaufman:

I have a weight problem, and my doctor refuses to give me diet pills. I don't understand why some doctors readily dispense such pills and others do not.

Answer:

It has been well said: It is food that makes one fat, not pills that make one thin. If there were a magic reducing pill that could be *safely* and consistently used, we would all know about it. So-called appetite suppressants can have undesirable and even dangerous side effects, and cannot be used for extended periods of time. Other pills, such as diuretics, have to do with water loss, not flesh loss, and have their own limitations and side effects, particularly with prolonged use.

Although various fad diets are capable of helping to reduce weight, the problem is what to do *after* the desired weight is attained. When that point is reached, the person is confronted with a basic fact: to maintain a certain weight requires dietary vigilance, helped by exercise.

Dear Dr. Kaufman:

How often is a tipped womb the cause of backache?

Answer:

A uterus that is tipped backward is normally seen in about 20 per cent of women. On rare occasions it may be responsible for backaches, the pain being characteristically worse during the premenstrual and early menstrual phase. Such pain is usually relieved by lying down. If there is some question as to whether the retroversion is causing the backache (and there generally *is* some question), the answer can be found by inserting a special pessary that holds the uterus forward. If there is complete relief of backache with the pessary in place, and a return to the backache when the pessary is removed and the uterus permitted to return to its original tipped position, then the cause and effect relationship is clarified.

Dear Dr. Kaufman:

For the past four months I have been staining for a day or two between periods and wonder if this is abnormal. Should I see a doctor? There is no pain.

Answer:

Vaginal spotting that occurs two weeks prior to a menstrual period is common and is usually attributed to ovulation (release of an egg from the ovary). It is not considered abnormal if the sequence of events is as described. To be certain, mark your calendar the next time this happens and note whether your next menstrual period comes just about 14 days later. If so, it is typical, though it need not recur every month (some women never experience the sign). If your staining occurs any time other than two weeks prior to menstruation, you should report it to your doctor for further investigation.

Dear Dr. Kaufman:

I was told that an iron supplement would be helpful because I have very heavy periods. However, my stomach gets upset from iron and I wonder what natural foods I can eat which will supplement my iron intake.

Answer:

Good food sources for iron are liver, meat, egg yolk, green leafy vegetables, peaches, raisins, prunes, and apricots.

Dear Dr. Kaufman:

I am 19 years old. My cycles are irregular and I often have prolonged light spotting between periods, which worries me. What could be the cause?

Answer:

A common cause for such spotting in young women is absence of ovulation. This condition creates a hormonal imbalance leading to sporadic spotting—an annoying, but not serious symptom. However, you should be examined in order to be certain that this is, in fact, the cause.

Dear Dr. Kaufman:

I have had vaginal itching on several occasions, but have never seen a doctor about it. What are the most likely causes?

Answer:

There are many possible causes. A common one seen nowadays is due to an allergic-type response to detergent soap, and to synthetic fabrics such as nylon, dacron, and others which, incidentally, also have a tendency to prevent good air circulation and keep a woman "wet." Itching may also develop as the result of sensitivity to douche powders, contraceptive jellies, and so-called feminine deodorant sprays. Hip-hugging pants also accentuate the irritating potential of any sensitizing matter in underpants.

Itching associated with a thick, white, cheesy discharge suggests a yeast (fungus, monilia) infection. A frothy discharge with odor suggests a trichomonas (parasitic) infection. In older women, itching is often associated with thinning and drying of the vaginal mucous membrane, due to estrogen deficiency. Less commonly, in older women, itching is also associated with degenerative diseases and other pathological conditions.

Dear Dr. Kaufman:

I have been greatly troubled with a copious clear discharge, almost to the point of having to wear a tampon. There is no irritation or itching, and several doctors who have examined me are unable to find any pathological causes. Do you have any thoughts or suggestions?

Answer:

The kind of discharge you describe—copious but clear and non-irritating—suggests a physiological cause. A frequently overlooked physiological cause is the use of contraceptive pills, which cause an increased secretion from the cervix. The sequential type of pill, with its relatively high estrogen content, is especially apt to produce this effect.

Another often unsuspected cause is unresolved sexual tension, a kind of chronic pelvic congestion from frequent stimulation alone. This cause can only be elicited by a careful history, as women usually do not associate the discharge as being either physiologic or sexually related.

Still another cause sometimes overlooked is a bacterial infection of the vagina that may produce discharge without irritation. Such infection (hemophilus) can be effectively treated in most cases with anti-bacterial vaginal cream or inserts.

Dear Dr. Kaufman:

I was told I had a fungus infection, and that this was the cause of my vaginal discharge and irritation. Is this serious? Is such a fungus the same as athlete's foot?

Answer:

A fungus infection of the vagina sounds far worse than it actually is. It is not serious, though it can be very annoying. It belongs in the yeast family, and is a different fungus from the one causing athlete's foot. There are several different kinds of medications that can be therapeutically effective.

Dear Dr. Kaufman:

A few months ago I developed a vaginal infection that the doctor said was due to trichomonas. He treated the infection, but it continues to recur. How can I keep it from coming back? My husband is getting very impatient!

Answer:

Your husband may be the carrier that is causing your recurrences. In such a situation, treatment directed toward both husband and the wife usually results in a cure.

Dear Dr. Kaufman:

Why is it that every time I take an antibiotic, I come down with a vaginal discharge and itch? This has happened to me three times in the past year.

Answer:

Antibiotics kill off normal protective vaginal bacteria, allowing yeast organisms, *if present*, free reign. It is the yeast (a form of fungus) that causes the vaginal discharge and itch. This recurring annoyance can be minimized or prevented by using anti-fungal vaginal medication at the same time that antibiotics are being taken.

Dear Dr. Kaufman:

Recently, every time I have intercourse I get a vaginal irritation and discharge. At other times I'm quite comfortable. My husband has no rashes or discomfort, but he is quite upset that intercourse should produce these symptoms. What could be the matter? We are in our twenties.

Answer:

It isn't that intercourse is producing the condition responsible for your vaginal discomforts, but rather that intercourse is aggravating an *existing* disorder, which is ordinarily quiescent. You probably have a latent vaginal infection from yeast or trichomonas which "lights up" from the friction of intercourse. An examination will disclose the true cause, and point the direction of cure.

Dear Dr. Kaufman:

I have noticed a lot of itching in the region of the pubic hair, and my doctor thinks it may be crab lice. Could you discuss this condition?

Answer:

Crab lice (pediculosis pubis) are not uncommon. They may be spread by sexual intercourse, but can also be spread by any close physical contact, or by infected blankets, clothing, pajamas, or toilet seats. The diagnosis is made by finding the lice in the pubic hairs. A magnifying lens and forceps are helpful in detaching and isolating the crab louse, usually difficult to find.

The crab louse is only 1 mm. long, barely visible to the naked eye. Under the low-power microscope, however, the louse looks like a giant crab with bristling hairs. There also may be ova (called nits) attached to the pubic hairs.

The preferred treatment is the use of a special lotion, used as a pubic hair shampoo. In order to avoid reinfection, all clothing that has been worn, blankets, and sheets must be laundered or dry cleaned. Toilet seats should also be cleaned thoroughly.

Interestingly, the pubic louse will not affect hairs in other parts of the body such as the scalp or armpits. A *different* louse inhabits those areas.

Dear Dr. Kaufman:

I have been plagued by herpes infections in the genital areas. It is very painful and distressing. Can anything be done to prevent this condition?

Answer:

Genital herpes, which is believed to be a viral disorder, is often difficult to treat at the time the patient has it. However, recurrences can often be aborted during the first 12-24 hours by the use of certain dyes combined with heat.

Dear Dr. Kaufman:

I have been bothered by little warts around the entrace of my vagina. What could this be due to?

Answer:

Vulvo-vaginal and anal "warts" have been variously called condylomata accuminata, papillomata, and venereal warts. The common, garden variety type (*not* truly venereal) is believed to be caused by a virus. Often there is associated vaginal inflammation, which may predispose. Treatment is usually by a chemical caustic which slowly dissolves the warts. Other forms of therapy include electrocautery (burning), cryosurgery (freezing), or, in extreme cases, surgical excision.

Dear Dr. Kaufman:

I have been using vaginal deodorant sprays for several weeks and find that they have lately become irritating. I wondered if this was a common complaint?

Answer:

After a long study and many reports about adverse reactions, the Food and Drug Administration has proposed that labels for all vaginal deodorant sprays carry warnings on possible problems such as you describe. Vaginal sprays, introduced in this country in 1966, are often advertised as "hygiene" sprays, but the FDA said it knew of no medical or hygienic benefits derived from them. The most frequent complaints are burns, irritation, discharge and rashes.

Aside from such unpleasant side effects, vaginal deodorant sprays do not appear to be the logical approach to "feminine hygiene." The genital area is not comparable to the underarm, and therefore the spray cannot possibly get into the vagina, nor would that be desirable.

Dear Dr. Kaufman:

When a woman douches, how far up does the fluid go? I mean, does it penetrate part way or far into the vagina, and does it reach the womb?

Answer:

Assuming that the woman is using the optimal position, which is lying on her back with the douche bag about two feet above the abdomen, the fluid will reach most of the vaginal surfaces. It can travel slightly into the cervix but not higher.

An interesting experiment was once made, in which women who were about to have a hysterectomy were asked to douche preoperatively with blue dye. (These women all had had several children, so that the cervix was not very tight.) Postoperatively, it could be demonstrated that in no instance did the dye reach the cavity of the uterus.

Dear Dr. Kaufman:

Is there any harm in simple douching during pregnancy? I use a small bulb syringe.

Answer:

This is precisely the kind of douche that should never be used during pregnancy, since with a hand syringe there is danger of air being injected into the uterus. There have been several maternal deaths reported due to air embolism, where the cause was vaginal douching with a bulb syringe. As for the use of an ordinary douche bag with multiple holed nozzle, some doctors permit its use during pregnancy while others do not.

Dear Dr. Kaufman:

For the past two years I have had a peculiar vaginal discharge. Sometimes it is whitish, and other times it is watery and clear. Should I consult a doctor? I am 15 years old.

Answer:

There is a common misunderstanding as to what constitutes an "abnormal" vaginal discharge. Actually, a little discharge, usually noted at the end of the day, is perfectly normal. The vagina, like the mouth, is never supposed to be completely dry. As long as the individual has no irritation or itching, and is not wet all day, the discharge cannot be described as being either abnormal or excessive. Your letter did not state whether you have begun to menstruate as yet. It is common for adolescent girls to develop a slight discharge during the months prior to the onset of menstruation.

Dear Dr. Kaufman:

I have a problem with urine leakage when I cough or sneeze. Please tell me if this is serious and what can be done to correct it.

Answer:

Urine leakage is certainly a most vexing problem. It is usually caused by relaxed muscles. A doctor must examine you to determine the proper therapy, whether it be special exercises to tighten the muscles, the insertion of a pessary (ring), or vaginal plastic surgery.

Dear Dr. Kaufman:

I am at my wits' end. About two months after my marriage I got cystitis, which went away but returns every few weeks. It causes painful and frequent urination. What should I do?

Answer:

There are two kinds of bladder inflammation. One is a purely mechanical irritation of the bladder neck, an area which happens to be separated from the vagina by only a thin band of tissue. It can be caused by frequent intercourse in newlyweds, hence the name "honeymoon cystitis" to describe it. However, this type usually subsides within a week or two.

The other kind of cystitis is due to actual bacterial infection of the bladder (and this can also be superimposed on the first type mentioned). It is therefore helpful to have a urine culture to find out if bacteria are responsible, and appropriate antibiotics can then be given.

Dear Dr. Kaufman:

Are urinary symptoms part of menopause? I am fifty-two and have had burning on urination for several months. My last period was over three years ago.

Answer:

The urethra, which is the canal leading from the bladder, is subject to the same thinning from lack of estrogen as the vaginal lining. When thinned this way there may be urinary frequency and discomfort when voiding. Such symptoms respond dramatically to the local application of estrogen to the vaginal area nearby, as well as to estrogen taken orally.

Dear Dr. Kaufman:

I am 60 years old and have had increasing vaginal irritation, especially if intercourse is attempted. Is this part of the aging process, or can something be done about it?

Answer:

Assuming that an examination reveals no pathogenic causes for vaginal irritation but does reveal a thin and reddened vaginal mucous membrane due to estrogen deficiency, the application of local estogenic cream can reverse the process in a matter of days, eliminating the irritation and making intercourse comfortable again. Usually it is necessary to re-apply the hormonal medication at intervals in order to keep the vaginal lining well nourished.

Dear Dr. Kaufman:

As soon as I returned from my honeymoon, I came down with all sorts of problems—a vaginal discharge, irritation, itching, and even urinary burning. I am certain that I could not have venereal disease, and yet I have never had anything like this before. What could be the trouble?

Answer:

You probably had organisms in the vagina, such as yeast or trichomonas, which were dormant until you began having intercourse; then they "kicked up." It is not an uncommon tale. The urinary complaints can be accounted for on the basis of mechanical irritation. Of course, you should be examined in order to check out these probabilities, and to institute proper treatment.

TWELVE

Change of Life

Dear Dr. Kaufman:

I have read and enjoyed your book on menopause. Most of the writings on menopause that I have noted have been in the past decade, or so it seems. Is there a reason for this?

Answer:

Survival into the postmenopausal years is a comparatively "recent" phenomenon. Back in ancient Rome, life expectancy was only about 23 years. By the 14th century it has risen to 33 years, and around the turn of the century it was only 48 or 49.

Today, a woman's life expectancy is closer to 75. Since the average age of menopause is around 50, a woman may live a third of her life after her menopause.

It is unfortunate that some writings have led women to believe that within their reach is a magic elixir which will keep them young forever. If a woman can separate the truth from half-truths and fiction, she has a chance at least for comfortable stability at this time of life.

Dear Dr. Kaufman:

What are the most common complaints that you hear from menopausal women?

Answer:

I missed a period for the first time—am I pregnant? My periods are very irregular—is it anything to worry about? I get hot and perspire a lot—and I can't sleep. I am irritable with my husband and children—can't anything be done? Sexual relations are painful—what can I do? And many more of a similar nature.

Dear Dr. Kaufman:

Is it true that humans are the only mammals whose females outlive their reproductive lives?

Answer:

True for all practical purposes. The only exception are cow elephants which live some 20 years after their last ovulation. There is also some evidence that female whales live well beyond reproductive age.

Dear Dr. Kaufman:

I have heard of the many benefits of estrogen therapy for menopausal symptoms but not too much about its limitations. Could you discuss the reliability of estrogen replacement therapy?

Answer:

Estrogen can relieve most of the physical discomforts of menopause that are due to estrogen deficiency and some of the associated emotional symptoms. Specifically, estrogen can definitely control hot flushes and associated sweating, perhaps the two most annoying symptoms. Local estrogen can also reverse vaginal thinning, eliminating a frequent cause of vaginal discomfort and painful intercourse in older women.

Estrogen will also relieve other menopausal complaints if the symptom is due to estrogen deficiency. It is often not possible to foretell until a trial with estrogen is undertaken. For instance, depression and insomnia are two common symptoms which may or may not be due to estrogen deficiency. When it is related, the hormone is helpful in relieving the complaint. The same is true of many other symptoms, any of which may be mimicked by non-hormonal factors.

In addition, estrogen is helpful in relieving the painful symptoms of osteoporosis (brittle bones) and some feel it can retard the progress of this poorly understood disorder. Whether estrogen "protects" a woman from heart ailments before menopause is debatable, although some circumstantial evidence seems to favor this theory.

It should be kept in mind that the relief of estrogen-related symptoms often enables a woman to cope with her remaining, unrelated complaints, whereas before hormone therapy the combination of symptoms could be overwhelming.

Estrogen has its limitations. It cannot slow the normal aging process. It has no direct effect upon female libido. Whether taken internally or rubbed on, estrogenic hormones will not prevent or eliminate wrinkles, nor will they end gray hair. Estrogens do not prevent the weight changes of middle age or keep the breasts forever youthful. And while they can produce artificial menstrual periods into advanced years, they cannot restore reproductive function.

Dear Dr. Kaufman:

I am 49 years old and lately my periods have become longer and much closer together. They are sometimes only two weeks apart, and I could continue to spot for 10 days. My doctor wants to investigate this further and seems concerned, but I am reluctant. My question is: isn't this a normal part of the expected "changes"?

Answer:

Although there are expected "changes," you are going in the wrong direction!

The normal pattern is for menstrual periods to become shorter (not longer), lighter (not heavier), further apart (not closer together), or to cease altogether. Undoubtedly your doctor is concerned because your pattern does not follow any of these avenues. Although the cause could still be nothing more than a "hormonal imbalance," physical causes should be carefully ruled out.

Dear Dr. Kaufman:

Why is it that so many women cease having intercourse after menopause?

Answer:

Perhaps the myth that older women can't have satisfactory sexual relations is so ingrained that many women *expect* their sex lives to taper off at the menopause. Others merely stop doing something which has always been disturbing or distasteful for them. And let's not overlook another reason: their husbands may not want to anymore.

Dear Dr. Kaufman:

What are some of the annoying side effects of estrogen therapy?

Answer:

Estrogen therapy can cause spotting, abnormally prolonged bleeding, nausea, breast tenderness, and fluid retention. It can increase the size of uterine fibroids, and although estrogen does not cause cancer, it may stimulate an already existing breast or genital cancer.

Dear Dr. Kaufman:

I am 49 and still get menstrual periods, though sometimes I skip a month. What are my chances of getting pregnant?

Answer:

Most doctors advise some form of contraception (it can be simple, like foam) until menstrual periods have ceased for a full year. However, as far as actual probabilities of pregnancy are concerned, a woman's fertility is almost zero by the time she is 50, even if she is still having menstrual periods.

Dear Dr. Kaufman:

I am going through menopause and am very depressed. However, several gynecologists and endocrinologists I have gone to told me that my depression has nothing to do with menopause, and that I need to see a psychiatrist to straighten out. I don't see what good a psychiatrist will do me. I think I'm a lost cause. Aren't hormones helpful in situations like mine?

Answer:

In situations like yours, where there is a note of desperation, all is not "lost" if you can possibly hold on to a sense of humor, which is, after all, a sense of balance. You have apparently decided in advance that your various doctors' suggestions will be fruitless. It's a good thing the doctors are not as pessimistic. Otherwise it would be like the story of the psychiatrist who says to his despondent patient: "Of course, I could cure you of your recurrent depression—except that, as you say, everything is so futile!"

Why not explore the possibility of relief with professional help, as has been suggested? Hormones (estrogen) will not help a depression which is not directly related to estrogen deficiency. The menopausal years are often burdensome and conducive to low moods from emotional causes.

Dear Dr. Kaufman:

If it is true that in the fifth decade or so a woman no longer has enough estrogen to menstruate, does it not follow that all such women need estrogen replacement?

Answer:

In my view, the mere fact that a woman does not have enough to menstruate is not a basis for menopausal treatment. It is the *rate* of estrogen decline that seems more important in the production of symptoms. My own therapeutic aim is to replace estrogen lack with a dosage adequate to control signs and symptoms of estrogen deficiency, but not necessarily so much as to restimulate the uterine lining to bleed.

Dear Dr. Kaufman:

Is estrogen being used now for the prevention of heart disease?

Answer:

Although there is no complete scientific proof as yet, some doctors believe that estrogens may act in a preventive manner regarding heart disease in women. More specifically, estrogens are usually recommended for women who have undergone removal of the ovaries before normal menopause. The hormone might also well be considered in women of any age group who have a family history of coronary heart disease or other factors that suggest a predisposition to coronary disease, such as obesity, diabetes, hypertension, or heavy smoking.

Dear Dr. Kaufman:

I have been told that I have a "senile" vaginal condition, though I am only 47 and still look and feel quite youthful. Please explain. My menopause was only two years ago.

Answer:

The term "senile" is most unfortunate. It has a connotation of creakiness associated with very advanced years—certainly not with someone who is 47. The term, as used medically, describes tissue rather than a person. The vaginal mucous membrane is very sensitive to estrogen deficiency and can show thinning and inflammation due to such lack, even though the woman feels fine. The medical term for this condition is "senile" or "atrophic" vaginitis. Happily, the condition is completely reversible by the simple local administration of estrogenic creams.

Dear Dr. Kaufman:

How common is pregnancy after menopause?

Answer:

Pregnancy during the late 40s and after is sufficiently uncommon to have occasioned a number of surveys. Almost all such reports mention the tremendous difficulties in obtaining exact menstrual histories and particularly in authenticating exact age.

One study concluded that, in general, pregnancy after age 47 is "highly unlikely," another that pregnancy in women over 50 is "extremely rare." A review of New York City vital statistics for 1940 to 1950 showed only 20 births by women 50 or over, among some 1,500,000 deliveries. One researcher reviewed the medical literature back to 1860; only 26 apparently authentic cases of women who had normal living babies after age 50 were found.

Nevertheless, medico-legal opinion tends to play it safe. For example, the British courts concluded that "we cannot pretend to fix the age at which pregnancy ceases to be possible and beyond which it cannot occur." The Common Law in the United States concurs, stating that a woman "is conclusively presumed to be capable of children until death. . ." In any event, a woman's fertility, unlike a man's does show a definite decline between ages 40 and 45, and a precipitous drop between 45 and 50, approaching zero at about 50.

Dear Dr. Kaufman:

What is the chief cause of depression in menopausal women?

Answer:

Psychologically, the menopausal woman often feels that she is losing her main purpose in life—whether this be her attractiveness (a fear of aging), her loss of reproductive function (which is lost at menopause), or her role as companion for her husband or mother to her grown children.

Depression may also be caused by a severe estrogen deficiency, and in such instances the symptom will be helped by estrogen replacement. On the other hand, when depression is caused by changes in life style and emotional upheaval, as with the reasons mentioned, estrogen alone will be of little value.

Dear Dr. Kaufman:

How often will variety in sexual techniques improve the sex life of a middle-aged couple?

Answer:

To say that such a couple need only apply a little more adventure in their lovemaking techniques is to oversimplify the problem. However, every so often, the resolving of certain sexual hangups helps a couple gain a new dimension in their physical closeness. Sometimes it takes a good deal of counseling to change deep-rooted notions that certain common sexual practices are "perverted."

Dear Dr. Kaufman:

Why are there so many sexual conflicts at the time of menopause?

Answer:

Menopause comes at a bad time of life—during middle age. And middle age brings its own physical and emotional problems, any of which can seriously affect sex. Menopause itself is a stark reminder to any woman that she is growing older, a depressing thought. Menopause also means loss of reproductive function. For those women who are childless, or who have fewer children than they had wanted, this can be a severe letdown, since there is no treatment that can restore fertility after menopause.

Other women become depressed over the "empty nest" syndrome. The children are grown, and mother is no longer needed. Or there may be problems with teenage children, many of whom are in their own state of turmoil, or are involved in a civil war with their parents. Depression, with accompanying diminished sexual drive and response, from causes such as this, cannot be expected to improve with hormonal therapy.

This is also the time of life when a woman's husband is likely to be busier than ever in business matters, paying less attention to his wife, who quickly interprets this as a lessening of his affection for her. And, indeed, this may be the case. Middle-aged men often have a feeling of discontent and futility at not having achieved everything they had hoped for, but such feelings are usually weathered *if* there are no serious rifts in the husband-wife relationship. It is no coincidence that divorce, which is common during the first few years of marriage, rises again during middle age. Sexuality is so sensitive a barometer that it literally shrivels if it is no longer desired. And this is the main reason why, in many marriages, sexual relations begin to dwindle during these critical years.

Often the wife has begun to lose her "appeal" through years of familiarity and habit. More likely, however, the marriage has simply ceased to be a vital force, and other interests have become more dominant. The middle-aged man is not unable to make love, but he may be unable to *give* love. His physical potency is there, but not his incentive to employ it and enjoy it. A vicious cycle follows: just when the husband is most in need of affirming his masculinity, his wife is plagued by doubts about her own desirability, with the result that neither gives the assurance the other requires. The husband may seek an affair with other women, or the wife with other men. And either event is very likely to deepen the rift to the point where only skilled marital counseling can begin to untangle the many strains.

Dear Dr. Kaufman:

Can estrogen therapy be effective for such complaints as insomnia, headache, fatigue and depression?

Answer:

Using a therapeutic trial of hormonal therapy, I have found that such symptoms are relieved to a greater or lesser extent in about 50 per cent of cases. Sometimes the results seem paradoxical. For example, I recall one woman who consulted me because of flushes, depression and headaches. After examination, I prescribed a trial of estrogen tablets. She reported some weeks later that her flushes had disappeared, her depression (in her words) had "lifted like a cloud," but the headaches persisted, indicating a different cause, and requiring different medication. In another patient, who had the identical complaints of flushes, depression and headache, estrogen therapy completely relieved the flushes and the headaches, but in her case the depression remained. In that instance, it was the depression that was unrelated to estrogen deficiency.

Dear Dr. Kaufman:

Can contraceptive pills be continued indefinitely to prevent menopausal symptoms? In other words, can menopause be postponed?

Answer:

In my opinion, there are several reasons for *not* continuing the pill indefinitely.

First, fertility falls so sharply after 45 that one no longer needs a potent contraceptive agent like the pill. Any of the simpler contraceptive methods are fully adequate at this time of life.

Second, menopause occurs anywhere between ages 40 and 55, after which there may still be adequate natural estrogenic production for many more years. One woman can have symptoms of estrogen deficiency at 42, another at 54 may as yet have no signs or symptoms. Since estrogen deficiency does not occur overnight, there is plenty of time to prevent the effect of such deficiency by medical evaluation every few months, and to give any one of several estrogenic preparations if needed.

Furthermore, continuing contraceptive pills indefinitely after fertility is over supplies a fixed amount of estrogen without knowing what the actual requirements are, and then only as a "package" with a potent progestin hormone. If continued, such pills can, indeed, induce "menstrual" periods into old age and, in this sense, menopause (the cessation of periods) is "prevented." However, in my own experience, most postmenopausal women are relieved when menstruation is over and are not at all eager to continue or renew monthly bleeding if given a choice.

Finally, and perhaps most important, the pill is often associated with irregular breakthrough bleeding or staining.

In young women, this is often casually managed by changing the dosage or product. But in women over 40, there is a rising natural incidence of pelvic disease which attaches much greater importance to any irregular staining. Because such staining may be wrongly interpreted as due to the pill, pelvic disease may be overlooked. For these various reasons, I believe there is little purpose in "postponing" menopause.

However, it should be added that not all doctors share these views. Some do prefer the continuation of contraceptive pills, particularly the sequential variety, well into the fifties and beyond.

Dear Dr. Kaufman:

Is it possible for estrogenic hormones to keep a woman young?

Answer:

Not really, but each woman has three different ages: her chronological age, marked by the calendar; her physiological (biological) age, which is the condition of her body; and her psychological age, which is how old she feels or acts.

I am reminded of a story about a 74-year-old woman who consulted a specialist in hormone therapy. After a thorough examination the doctor said, "Madame, you're in good shape, but I simply can't make you any younger." Replied the woman, "Don't worry about that. Just let me keep getting older!"

About 30 percent of women pass through menopause easily, age gracefully, and continue to enjoy life and sex into advanced years. But a majority of women run into varying degrees of trouble with postmenopause and estrogen deficiency, and do require help.

Dear Dr. Kaufman:

Is there a male menopause? My husband, who is 55, thinks there is. I have heard conflicting viewpoints.

Answer:

The answer is both yes and no! Let me explain. I say no, because the term itself is an absurdity. Menopause means cessation of menstrual periods which men, of course, don't have. Nor is there an abrupt decline in hormonal function in men, in contrast to the pattern observed in many women.

However, the same kind of emotional symptoms that have often been associated with female menopause may overtake men of comparable age. Nervousness, diminished sexual drive, sleep disturbances, irritability, fatigue, loss of self-confidence, and so on. Many psychiatrists believe that the depression overtaking many middle-aged men is largely one that has to do with unfulfillment, not to hormonal change.

THIRTEEN

Benign Growths

Dear Dr. Kaufman:

Is it true that fibroid tumors of the womb are common? How early in life can they occur? I am 26, and my doctor said I have a small fibroid.

Answer:

Fibroids, which are benign fibromuscular growths of the uterine wall, are indeed common. However, they do not occur before puberty; apparently estrogenic stimulation is necessary. They are also rare in the late teens and even in the early twenties, being more common in the thirties and forties. The trend is reversed at the menopause. At that time fibroids begin to shrink to about a third their size. Small fibroids that produce no symptoms require no treatment.

About one out of five women over 35 has at least one fibroid. Usually they cause no symptoms, and a woman is not even aware she has them. When they are bothersome, the symptoms usually relate to menstruation—either heavier periods or other menstrual abnormalities. The position of the fibroid is important in relation to symptoms. A large one at the surface may produce no effects, but one projecting into the womb, even if very small, can cause profuse bleeding. A large fibroid on the back of the womb may cause rectal pain, pain during intercourse, or constipation. A large fibroid on the front of the uterus can simulate a pregnancy and cause urinary frequency and urgency.

Dear Dr. Kaufman:

One doctor told me I have a fibroid growth on my uterus the size of an orange, and it need only be watched, but another doctor said it was the size of a grapefruit and should be removed. Now I don't know what to do. (Both examined me the same week.)

Answer:

It is entirely understandable that you should be confused, as you have been given conflicting opinions with different recommendations. Reference to fruit to describe the size of a tumor growth can lead to even more confusion. On most hospital records, doctors report the size of pelvic tumors in terms of centimeters or pregnancy size—for example, an 8- or 10-week gestation. In that way, everyone understands what size is meant.

Since you have two conflicting opinions, I would suggest you see a gynecologist for a third opinion. Your letter does not mention your age, whether you have had children, or any symptoms connected with the fibroid. These, rather than size alone, may be of importance in reaching a decision.

Dear Dr. Kaufman:

I was told I had a sebaceous cyst on the vulva. It is small, about the size of a jelly bean. I can feel it when I bathe, but it doesn't really bother me. Any cause for alarm?

Answer:

Sebaceous cysts of the vulva occur often in the hairy region of the labia majora. When infected, such small cysts may cause great concern to the patient, who notices the sudden appearance of an enlarging "lump" and may fear cancerous growth. Surgical intervention is only occasionally necessary, chiefly for cosmetic reasons, or for the relief of persistent discomfort from infection.

Dear Dr. Kaufman:

During a routine checkup, my doctor told me I had some cysts on my cervix and proceeded to burn them off. I must admit it was painless, but was taken aback by the discovery. I do recall having had a cervical erosion many months ago, but that was all cleared up. Could you tell me where such cysts come from? Are they harmful?

Answer:

In all probability you had some "Nabothian" cysts, which are blobs on the cervix, the end result of a chronic "burned-out" infection. They are harmless, and are easily obliterated by burning with electrocautery, at which time the retained fluid they contain runs out.

Dear Dr. Kaufman:

Could you name different types of ovarian cysts? Why is it that some can be treated with medication, while others require surgery?

Answer:

When an ovary, normally small and rubbery, becomes swollen like a balloon or filled with a liquid substance, it is known as an ovarian cyst. There are many types, too numerous to go into great detail. However, two types related to hormonal function are "follicular cysts" (when they result from over-accumulation of follicular fluid), and "corpus luteum cysts" (which result from undue swelling of the shell from which the egg was extruded). Such hormonally-related cysts generally subside spontaneously without any treatment, and no surgery is necessary unless there is significant internal bleeding or twisting of the cyst.

Another common type of cyst is called a "dermoid" and is most interesting, since it is composed of embryonic elements, often including hair and teeth! The latter can be spotted on an x-ray film. Such cysts are usually benign, but should be removed, since they also contain a heavy, waxy material and have a tendency to grow larger and to twist.

Another type, also common, is called a "chocolate cyst" due to dark brown material found within. The brown color is due to old blood, caused by monthly bleeding within the cyst itself. The condition is actually the result of endometriosis, wherein uterine lining cells are oddly found within the cyst and "bleed" each month, just as though they were still in the uterus. Such cysts are generally large enough and sufficiently uncomfortable to warrant surgery.

An ovarian cyst may require surgery because of how it feels (solid-feeling, enlarged ovaries demand exploration); or because of size alone (a cyst which is persistently over 3 inches or so), or because of the symptoms it may cause (usually pain). In all cases, but particularly in older women, the possibility of a malignancy is in the doctor's mind in evaluating each case.

If operated on, many cysts do not require complete sacrifice of the entire ovary and, indeed, in younger women who have not completed their families, endometrial cysts and dermoids are often "resected," meaning that the cyst portion is removed, leaving behind some normally functioning ovarian tissue. Conservative surgery is especially likely when the cysts involve both ovaries. Of course, there is always the chance that such cysts will recur in the future, but in younger women that risk is usually preferred to removal. In older women, ovarian surgery is seldom conservative, since childbearing function is usually complete, and the risk of ovarian malignancy is higher in that age group.

Dear Dr. Kaufman:

I have had a painless, grape-sized lump just within the opening of my vagina, toward the right side. It has been there for about two years. Once it swelled to the size of a small plum for a few days, then it went back to its former size. I was told that it was harmless and to leave it alone, but I am still concerned. Can't it be easily removed?

Answer:

You have described a cyst of one of your Bartholin glands (there is one on each side). These glands provide some lubrication but they may swell due to blockage of the duct from trauma or infection. Small Bartholin cysts that cause no discomfort are usually left alone. When persistently large, or when the cyst becomes infected and painful (Bartholin ab-
s eatment is surgical, usually by laying open the cyst
revent future clogging.

Dear Dr. Kaufman:

What is pelvic inflammatory disease? A doctor at a clinic I went to mentioned this as the reason for my pains. What are the causes of this disorder?

Answer:

There is a direct pathway from the opening to the womb into the abdominal cavity. Normally, there are protective mechanisms against the ascent of harmful bacteria, such as a "plug" of mucus in the cervix, and tiny hairs in the lining of the tubes that maintain a sweeping motion toward the uterus. Despite these body defenses against invasion of bacteria, there may be a bacterial beachhead established, the two most aggressive ones being gonorrhea and streptococcal infection.

Gonorrhea ascends directly into the uterus and tubes, whereas a strep infection attacks the tubes by roundabout veins and lymphatics. In any event, these or other organisms can produce a chronic tubal infection or pelvic abscess with resultant pain, disability, and sterility. The chronic infection or inflammation is known as pelvic inflammatory disease.

Dear Dr. Kaufman:

I have been plagued by pelvic pain for several years and have been examined by many doctors. Apparently the cause is not clear. Is there any way of finding out once and for all what the cause of my pain is, or must I assume that it is all in my head (as some doctors have told me).

Answer:

There is a way of finding out whether there is any physical cause for this chronic discomfort. It is a minor surgical procedure known as a laparoscopy, whereby the doctor can look directly into the pelvis and see all the organs. That way, it can be determined whether there is any physical basis for your pains.

Dear Dr. Kaufman:

I have vaginal staining only after intercourse. Actually, I notice the staining on my diaphragm when I remove it the next day. What could be wrong?

Answer:

Vaginal bleeding, or staining, that occurs after intercourse is usually caused by some local condition such as an inflammation of the neck of the uterus (cervical erosion), or a polyp (benign fleshy growth). A checkup and Pap smear are in order, to determine the exact cause of the spotting and the means of eliminating it.

Dear Dr. Kaufman:

I go to a clinic and have been told that I have an erosion of my cervix. Is this common? What causes it? Is the condition serious?

Answer:

Cervical erosions are indeed common. The word "erosion" does sound rather scary, but it needn't be, for the condition is essentially benign. An erosion might be described as a "raw" area on the neck of the womb, caused by local bacteria which produce a different type of surface cell. Since the cervix should always be kept in healthy condition, erosions should be treated by appropriate office therapy—cautery, local medications, or "freezing." Any erosion that fails to heal properly requires further medical investigation.

Dear Dr. Kaufman:

What is cervicitis? Can it prevent pregnancy? Can it be cured?

Answer:

Cervicitis is a low-grade infection of the cervix caused, in most cases, by local bacteria. The condition is quite common, and when it is chronic a thick secretion may result that can interfere with fertility by blocking sperm. A special test can disclose if this is the case.

Cervicitis can be cured. The most common treatment is by electrocautery, a painless burning process (there are no pain fibers for heat or cold in the cervix). Other modes of therapy include medicated suppositories, antibiotics, and cryosurgery (freezing).

Dear Dr. Kaufman:

What is a polyp? My doctor said he removed one from my womb (not in the hospital).

Answer:

A polyp is a soft fleshy growth that can occur anywhere in the body. In your case, it was probably in the cervix. When small, cervical polyps can be removed in the office without any difficulty. Such growths are almost never malignant.

Polyps can also develop high up in the cavity of the womb. In that location they cannot be seen except by means of x-ray, but their presence may be suspected from the woman's history or symptoms. A minor operative procedure in the hospital is required for the removal of polyps within the womb.

FOURTEEN

But Is It Cancer?

Dear Dr. Kaufman:

What is the origin of the word "cancer?"

Answer:

It derives from the Latin: crab. The term was first used by Greek and Roman physicians familiar with breast cancer, which typically had a claw-like appearance of the veins extending from the tumor.

Dear Dr. Kaufman:

My mother had breast cancer, and I understand that my risk is greater because of this family history. I am 33 years old and have two children. How much greater are my risks, and what other conditions play a role in increasing or decreasing such risks of breast cancer?

Answer:

The daughter of a woman with breast cancer has about twice the average risk of developing this disease, and the sister of a breast cancer patient has about 2½ times the risk.

Other factors appear to be less dominant. For example, there appears to be a slightly higher than average risk in women with fibrocystic breast disease, in childless women, in women with underactive thyroids, and in women who live in cold rather than warm climates and have a high socio-economic status.

There are also conditions which *decrease* the risk of breast cancer. Women who have had their first child before age 25 have about half the average risk. The risk appears to diminish still further below that age, so that women who have had a child before age 21 (especially before age 18) have only one-third to one-quarter the average risk.

Dear Dr. Kaufman:

I would be interested in knowing how the Pap smear originated.

Answer:

Dr. George Papanicolaou (1883-1962) became convinced that the vaginal smear was a reliable indicator of malignant change, and published his first report on the technique in 1928. That paper went almost unnoticed! For the next twelve years, Papanicolaou's investigations centered on endocrinology, until Dr. Joseph C. Hinsey, then Dean of Cornell Medical College, read his paper and encouraged him to resume his early research.

In 1942, Dr. Papanicolaou developed a staining procedure for uterine cancer cells, and in 1943 published with Dr. Herbert F. Traut a monograph entitled *Diagnosis of Uterine Cancer by the Vaginal Smear.* The potential significance of the procedure for the diagnosis of pre-invasive cancer immediately aroused the interest of the medical profession and the results were soon confirmed by others.

After the acceptance of the vaginal smear technique, Dr. Papanicolaou expanded his studies to the detection of cancer from cells shed from the lung, esophagus, stomach, rectum and bladder. He worked long hours in his laboratories at Cornell and also at home, assisted by his wife. Even in his seventies he continued to teach medical students, and published a steady succession of books and articles.

The original paper referred to (1928) was called *New Cancer Diagnosis.* It begins as follows: "I will only give a report of some work of mine which may have some bearing on the diagnosis of certain malignant tumors, especially those of the female genital tract. This work was started about two and one-half years ago in the spring of 1925 . . ." And in his summary, Dr. Papanicolaou said, "We have a new diagnostic method for certain malignant tumors especially of the female genital tract . . . I think this work will be carried a little further. . . I think that some method can and will be developed in the future."

Modest even then, as he was the rest of his life, Dr. "Pap," as he affectionately became known, was the great pioneer who originated the test that bears his name throughout the world.

Dear Dr. Kaufman:

Is the Pap smear used for anything besides cancer detection?

Answer:

Yes. The routine Pap test, which consists of the microscopic examination of cells taken from the vagina and cervix, is of course best known as a test to detect cancer of the womb (most particularly the cervix) in its earliest, pre-cancerous stage. However, smears from the vagina and cervix can also aid in estimating hormonal production, and determining the presence of common vaginal infections.

Dear Dr. Kaufman:

What are the most common sites of pelvic cancer in women?

Answer:

Statistical reports indicate that at present the most common pelvic cancer in white women involves the uterine lining (endometrium). The next most frequent site is cancer of the ovary, and the third most common area is the cervix. In black women, cervical cancer is most frequent, followed by cancer of the ovary, then cancer of the uterine lining.

The most ominously unchanged statistic concerns cancer of the ovary; the over-all incidence today is the same as it was some 25 years ago.

Dear Dr. Kaufman:

I understand that the Pap test has been very useful in detecting *pre*malignant changes in the cervix, resulting in a lowered incidence of cervical cancer. Has there been comparable progress with ovarian cancer?

Answer:

Unfortunately, no. Cancer of the ovary has been properly called the "silent" cancer because it is very difficult to detect in its early stages. Of all gynecological malignancies, ovarian cancer has the worst prognosis, and this is mainly due to late diagnosis. Moreover, ovarian cancer often mimicks a host of other disorders, such as gastro-intestinal disease, thus further delaying diagnosis, which is difficult at best.

Dear Dr. Kaufman:

I am 41 years old and was advised to have a curettage (D&C) for abnormal bleeding. I asked whether the doctor could get an immediate report from the laboratory as to whether there was an evidence of malignancy. He said no, it would take a day or two. Isn't there something called a frozen section that gives results in a few minutes?

Answer:

Frozen sections are often helpful in reaching a diagnosis, but unfortunately not in the case of uterine curettings. The tissue in the case of a D&C reaches the pathologist too "mashed up" for such a test, and must be painstakingly processed for definitive and accurate diagnosis in most cases.

Dear Dr. Kaufman:

I have heard that poor women have a higher risk of cervical cancer than their more affluent neighbors. Is this true?

Answer:

It is true that poor women, who are unfortunately the least likely to take advantage of cervical smear tests, are the most vulnerable to cervical cancer. Fear and apathy are the two greatest barriers to acceptance of such (Pap) smears among these women. Many women still fear gynecological examinations, especially if such examinations or tests could lead to surgery.

Dear Dr. Kaufman:

I have had a chronic herpes infection of my external genitals and have read that herpes may be related to cancer. Is this true? It has worried me greatly.

Answer:

Some studies have shown that of women with genital herpes, a higher percentage have evidence of premalignant or malignant changes in the cervix, as compared to women without genital herpes. Also, genital herpes and cervical cancer have similar epidimeologic features. They both occur most frequently in the lower socio-economic groups, and among women who begin sexual activity early in life.

Dear Dr. Kaufman:

I am using estrogenic cream for burning in the vaginal area. I have recently read that estrogens have caused cancer in animals. Do you think that it is safe for people to use?

Answer:

Although estrogens in massive doses have produced cancer in certain susceptible experimental animals, such cancer has not been produced in animals more closely resembling humans, such as the monkey. More important, estrogens have never been shown to produce cancer in humans, although diethylstilbestrol (DES) has been associated with vaginal or cervical cancer in occasional *offspring* of women who had received this particular drug during their early pregnancy.

Estrogens have been used for various conditions for some 30 years, and there has been no significant change in the incidence of female genital or breast cancer. Incidentally, you are using a *local* form of estrogen, very little of which is absorbed into the body.

Dear Dr. Kaufman:

What is the incidence of breast cancer?

Answer:

Breast cancer, the most common malignancy in women, will develop in 6 per cent of all women. Cancer of the breast is most frequent in older women, 75 per cent occurring in women over forty.

Dear Dr. Kaufman:

My 15-year-old daughter has been menstruating regularly for one year, and now has some prolonged vaginal bleeding. I know for a fact that I have never had any hormones during my pregnancy with her and therefore this could not be one of those cases of cancer in a young girl's genital tract associated with maternal hormonal ingestion. Do you think it is necessary for this young girl to be examined or can we assume that her bleeding is just due to some hormonal imbalance?

Answer:

She definitely should be examined. In a thorough review of cases involving young girls who have vaginal or cervical cancer, occasionally negative histories have been encountered, which suggests that factors other than maternal hormonal ingestion are operative in such tumor formation. Therefore, prolonged vaginal bleeding in young girls can no longer be assumed to be due solely to hormonal imbalance (though this is still the most probable cause), and such girls should have a pelvic examination whether or not there is a history of maternal hormonal intake.

Dear Dr. Kaufman:

I have read that cancer of the cervix is very rare in virginal women and is almost unheard-of in nuns. Is this true?

Answer:

There is little doubt from the studies conducted that the incidence is indeed very low. In one such survey there was a review of medical records of several nunneries in Quebec, Canada, over a period of 20 years. The author could not find a single case of cervical cancer. In fact, the rarity of the condition prompted a report in a medical journal, the *International Journal of Gynecology and Obstetrics,* entitled "A Case of Carcinoma of the Cervix in a Virgin."

Dear Dr. Kaufman:

What predisposes to the development of cancer of the inside of the womb?

Answer:

Cancer of the endometrium (womb lining) is more common in single women, childless women, menopausal or postmenopausal women, and particularly if there is any associated diabetes, obesity, or history of not stopping menstruation until past fifty.

There is also a somewhat increased incidence of this disease in young women between 18 and 25 who are obese, have menstrual abnormalities, and are unable to become pregnant.

Dear Dr. Kaufman:

Is it true that cancer is a common cause of vaginal bleeding after the menopause?

Answer:

Yes. Any bleeding one year or longer after menopause is always viewed with the greatest suspicion, since cancer of the uterus is one of the common causes of such bleeding in this age group. The physician will want to investigate such bleeding very carefully.

FIFTEEN

When Surgery Is Needed

Dear Dr. Kaufman:

One hears a great deal about unnecessary surgery being performed on women, and I wondered how a woman could be sure that surgery is really needed. In my own case, I had a hysterectomy at the age of 42 for fibroids with much hemorrhaging, but I have spoken to friends who have also had hysterectomies for apparently non-emergency reasons.

Answer:

Whenever there is any doubt in a patient's mind about the validity of a recommendation such as a hysterectomy, she has the option of seeking one or more additional opinions from other gynecologists of her own choosing. There is no question but that truly unnecessary surgery is to be deplored. However, as you yourself have noted, each case is obviously different and must be judged on its own merits.

Hysterectomy may be necessitated by a variety of conditions. Certainly a cancer anywhere in the reproductive tract is an indication. In the case of uterine fibroids, hysterectomy is usually advised when one of the following prevails: (1) recurrent, profuse periods (often from fibroid pressure into the uterine cavity), unresponsive to hormonal medication; (2) fibroids that have reached the size of a 3-3½-month pregnancy, particularly if there are any signs of pressure on other organs, such as the urinary tract; and (3) a sudden, marked increase in growth of fibroids, indicating the rare possibility of malignant change.

There is also a conservative operation for uterine fibroids known as "myomectomy" wherein such tumors are removed, attempting to leave the uterus intact. This is done in women who are eager to retain their childbearing function, but where the tumors seem to interfere with the ability to conceive, or cause repeated miscarriage.

Other conditions where hysterectomy *might* be advised are: (1) extensive pelvic endometriosis with disabling symptoms in a woman whose childbearing desire is complete and in whom conservative (hormonal) therapy has either been unsuccessful or is medically undesirable; (2) pelvic inflammatory disease with recurrent incapacity, where reproductive function is over or obviously compromised by the disease, and there is need to "clean out" the pelvis to effect a permanent cure; (3) when it is necessary to remove both ovaries for disease, it is best to remove the uterus at the same time, or it remains a useless organ subject to future disorders; (4) in certain vaginal plastic operations in older women for prolapse (herniation; bulge) of the uterus, bladder, or rectum. Here the uterus, which may be quite normal, is often purposely removed during the vaginal operation in order to facilitate the end result—the prevention of future prolapse.

There are also conditions where a "D&C (dilatation and curettage) or other similar biopsy procedure reveals the presence in the uterus of tissue which is believed to have a premalignant potential (adenomatous or atypical hyperplasia). The persistence of such tissue, particularly in the presence of recurrent abnormal bleeding, usually warrants a hysterectomy as a "preventive" measure. A hysterectomy can also be a life-saving measure in the rare instance of uncontrollable bleeding following a delivery, if all conservative measures fail.

Surgery for ovarian disease is also highly individualized. In women of childbearing age, an ovarian cyst (soft, fluid-containing tumor) which is 3 inches in diameter, and persists in such size, will probably warrant exploration. Cysts that are substantially larger, or solid ovarian tumors of *any* size, should be explored without awaiting further observations. In older women, ovaries gradually shrink after menopause and should normally become non-palpable 3-5 years postmenopausally. Ovarian cancer is one of the most insidious of female diseases and has become the leading killer of women from gynecologic malignancy. Early detection can be life saving.

Surgery for disorders of the fallopian tubes is also performed under special circumstances. An ectopic pregnancy (lodged in the tube) usually requires removal of the affected tube, though occasionally it is possible to remove the pregnancy while preserving the tube. Probably the most common operations on fallopian tubes are in certain infertility cases, where a careful investigation has shown all factors to be normal except for closure or severe narrowing of the tubes, as proven by endoscopy (direct visualization). An appropriate tubal reconstruction procedure is done in order to improve chances of conception.

Dear Dr. Kaufman:

I need an operation on my ovary and am concerned that my scar doesn't show, since I am a dancer by profession. I understand that certain scars are almost invisible. Is this true?

Answer:

Yes, the so-called "bikini" incision, which is at the upper level of the pubic hairline, is popular for that reason. When the hair regrows, the scar is almost invisible. It is a commonly used incision for pelvic operations, and has other advantages. Aside from its cosmetic value, there is much less tendency for wound disruption with this type of incision. However, it does not give as much room as a vertical incision, and the latter is often prefered when removing good-sized tumors.

Dear Dr. Kaufman:

I wish all gynecologists could undergo at least one major operation themselves in order to know what it feels like to be really sick. I'll never forget my first few days after surgery, with fever, pain, even a cough. Every time I coughed, I was sure I would bust a stitch. All my doctor did was to look at my chart and tell me I was doing very well!

Answer:

There is no question that a doctor who has personally experienced an operation or serious illness is at least better able to understand what some of his patients go through, and it may make him more empathic. The operation may have gone very well, but for the patient it's the crumbs in the bed that are of major importance at a given moment.

Some surgeons have, in fact, been through surgery or major illnesses, and they are not likely to forget it when it comes to sympathizing with sick patients.

Dear Dr. Kaufman:

Some of my friends who have had a hysterectomy say that the gynecologist also removed their appendix, while others left it in. What determines the decision?

Answer:

Although appendicitis is not common in older age groups, it may occur. Therefore, some doctors like to remove the appendix preventively—"as long as they're in the neighborhood"—provided the hysterectomy procedure is uncomplicated. Others prefer to leave the appendix alone, unless it looks diseased. Whatever the feelings are, any intention to remove the appendix should be discussed preoperatively.

Dear Dr. Kaufman:

I have a cyst on one of my ovaries, which hasn't bothered me. However, my doctor said it should be removed because it could "twist" at any time, producing an emergency situation. How often do ovarian cysts twist?

Answer:

Often enough to be included in well-known gynecological emergencies. However, it depends upon the type of cyst, as well as the size, heavier cysts having a greater tendency to twist.

Dear Dr. Kaufman:

The word hysterectomy is used to describe removal of the uterus, according to my understanding. Could you tell me the derivation of the word?

Answer:

Hysterectomy and hysteria come from the same source, which is "hyster," meaning uterus. The word "hysterical" reminds us that the association of the uterus with the emotions dates back to ancient times. It persists in common myths, such as the removal of the uterus (hysterectomy) leading to insanity, loss of sexual pleasure, etc.

Dear Dr. Kaufman:

I am 29 years old. I have been told by one doctor that I have a cyst on an ovary, and by another doctor that my ovaries are normal. I am thoroughly confused, and wondered what you would advise.

Answer:

Perhaps both doctors are right! It is possible you have a type of cyst (soft enlargement) that swells just before a menstrual period, when there is general congestion, and then recedes after the period is over. Check back as to the time of your cycle when each doctor examined you. Just as the breasts can become swollen premenstrually, so, too, can one or both ovaries. In such cases the important thing is to note whether the ovarian swelling is merely transient or continuing. By the way, if the time of your cycle does not account for this discrepancy, I would advise seeking a third opinion, but be sure to go after a menstrual period, when there is least congestion.

Dear Dr. Kaufman:

I am 43 years old and need a hysterectomy. One doctor told me he would definitely try to leave my ovaries in, to preserve my ovarian function and prevent premature menopause. However, another doctor told me he would definitely remove them in order to eliminate the possibility of ovarian malignancy in the future. I then went to a third doctor, who was noncommittal. Why is there so much controversy regarding this subject?

Answer:

The reason for the controversy is that no one has a crystal ball that can accurately predict the future course of developments for any woman. There are only statistics to go by. If the ovaries are left in there is, of course, a chance of future ovarian cancer or some other disease of these organs. Since ovarian function declines significantly in most women after 40–45, many surgeons suggest the removal of the ovaries at the time of hysterectomy, and this makes good sense.

Dear Dr. Kaufman:

Is there such a thing as complete absence of the vagina? If so, can this be corrected?

Answer:

Such a condition does exist. Various operations have been devised for correcting the anomaly, with varying degrees of success. The most dramatic instance recently reported in the popular press is an actual graft from mother to daughter, in which the mother needed to have her uterus removed and consented to have her vagina removed as well, to be grafted to her 27-year-old daughter who happened to lack this organ completely. The graft apparently took successfully.

Dear Dr. Kaufman:

After total hysterectomy, is there any need for routine annual Pap smears?

Answer:

If the hysterectomy was done for benign disease, then the only reason for doing a Pap smear would be for the possibility of cancer of the vagina. Although the incidence of this disease is low, some doctors will do smears at intervals for this possibility. Of course, if the patient had a hysterectomy for a malignancy, then routine follow-up Pap smears every few months are important.

Dear Dr. Kaufman:

One of my friends had her uterus removed through the abdomen. Another friend about the same age (in her fifties) had hers removed through the vagina. What determines the choice?

Answer:

Large tumors usually require the abdominal incision, since they are simply too large to be removed through the vagina. The abdominal approach is also used if there are other conditions present that require attention, such as suspected tumors of the ovaries, or if there is a known cancer of the uterus.

The uterus may be removed through the vagina (if it is not too large) when there is a relaxation of the bladder or rectal walls which need repair at the same time, or if the uterus itself has protruded through the vagina (dropped womb).

Dear Dr. Kaufman:

Is it true that a woman usually becomes fat and flabby after a hysterectomy?

Answer:

Not unless she eats too much. A gain in weight after any operation may be due to the fact that the person feels better as a result of the operation. An additional cause is the inactivity caused by the operation.

Dear Dr. Kaufman:

What happens if the ovaries are removed surgically, but the uterus is left in place? Does the woman still menstruate?

Answer:

No, the woman would not have any more menstrual periods since it is the ovaries that produce the hormones that cause the uterus to bleed each month. Ordinarily, however, when both ovaries have to be removed, the uterus is also removed, since it would otherwise remain a useless organ, subject to disease.

Dear Dr. Kaufman:

I am 51 years old, with menopause three years ago. I have had a small fibroid tumor on my womb for a number of years. Lately it seems to have gotten larger, according to my doctor. He is planning to operate if it continues to grow. How common is this condition?

Answer:

Uterine fibroids do not normally grow after the menopause; on the contrary, most fibroids shrink considerably at that time of life due to diminished hormonal production. Therefore, if it is growing, an operation would be the proper procedure, as advised. Sometimes what is thought to be a fibroid on the womb turns out to be a growth on an ovary. In either case, it would be important to investigate.

Dear Dr. Kaufman:

My doctor said that I had a prolapse of the vagina and said it was something like a sock turned inside out. I can feel a bulge when I'm up and around, and it also interferes with intercourse. Surgical repair was suggested, but I am wondering whether such surgery would interfere with having a good sex life afterward.

Answer:

A prolapse (herniation) of the vaginal tissues is not uncommon and a gynecologist can do the necessary surgical repair to correct it. Many different kinds of repair are possible without destroying the possibility of continued sexual enjoyment.

There is one type of complete herniation which is sometimes treated in the elderly by closing off the vagina surgically. However, such a procedure is only contemplated if it is certain that the woman, usually a widow, has no intention of resuming sexual relations. Your situation is obviously different.

Dear Dr. Kaufman:

I am 28 years old and have one child. Recently I had a bout of pain on my right side, and the doctor couldn't decide between an inflamed tube and appendicitis. It turned out to be the tube, and fortunately I did not need surgery. Even though I was the patient, I couldn't help sympathizing with the doctor, who obviously had a dilemma that had to be decided one way or another. Do you have problems like that frequently?

Answer:

Well, I can recall one for the books. The patient was your age and also had one child. She had severe pains on the left, away from the appendix, but that didn't make the problem any easier. I thought she had a left ectopic (tubal) pregnancy, another doctor thought she had a left twisted ovarian cyst, and still another doctor thought she had a degenerating uterine fibroid. At operation she turned out to have all three!

Index